REMEMBERING LOVE: A CAREGIVER'S GUIDE TO DEMENTIA AND ALZHEIMER'S

UNDERSTAND SIGNS & SYMPTOMS, MANAGE EMOTIONAL & FINANCIAL CHALLENGES, LEARN SKILLS TO CARE FOR AND COMMUNICATE WITH YOUR LOVED ONE

MARY ANN MARTIN

© **Copyright 2023 - All rights reserved.**

The content contained within this book may not be reproduced, duplicated or transmitted without direct written permission from the author or the publisher.

Under no circumstances will any blame or legal responsibility be held against the publisher, or author, for any damages, reparation, or monetary loss due to the information contained within this book, either directly or indirectly.

Legal Notice:

This book is copyright protected. It is only for personal use. You cannot amend, distribute, sell, use, quote or paraphrase any part, or the content within this book, without the consent of the author or publisher.

Disclaimer Notice:

Please note the information contained within this document is for educational and entertainment purposes only. All effort has been executed to present accurate, up to date, reliable, complete information. No warranties of any kind are declared or implied. Readers acknowledge that the author is not engaged in the rendering of legal, financial, medical or professional advice. The content within this book has been derived from various sources. Please consult a licensed professional before attempting any techniques outlined in this book.

By reading this document, the reader agrees that under no circumstances is the author responsible for any losses, direct or indirect, that are incurred as a result of the use of the information contained within this document, including, but not limited to, errors, omissions, or inaccuracies.

For Hilda and Mary

CONTENTS

Introduction	vii
1. Dementia Unveiled: Types, Stages, Symptoms, and Progression	1
2. Decoding Medical Jargon: Bridging the Gap between Caregivers and Healthcare Providers	16
3. Grasping the Basics: Understanding Medical Treatments for Dementia	26
4. Finding the Right Words: Successful Communication with Dementia Patients	38
5. The Daily Routine: Practical Skills for Caregiving	50
6. Decoding Dementia Behaviors: A Compassionate Approach	62
7. Navigating the Emotional Labyrinth: Strategies for Dealing with Stress, Guilt, and Burnout	71
8. Finding Strength in Numbers: Building Your Support Network	85
9. Making Cents of It All—Tackling Financial Challenges of Dementia Care	99
10. Safeguarding the Journey: Legal Guide to Dementia Care	110
11. Farewell, But Not Goodbye: Navigating the Journey Beyond Caregiving	120
Share Your Experience with Another Caregiver	129
Afterword	131
Glossary	135
Bibliography	139

INTRODUCTION

Dementia caregiving is a daunting task full of uncertainty and, at times, overwhelming worry. However, in those quiet moments, when everything seems to fade slowly into the background and all that is left is you and your loved one, the truth about caregiving hits home like a tsunami filled with complex emotions and unanswered questions. In these moments, we realize, in the deepest recesses of our hearts, the monumental impact of dementia and our role as caregivers. We realize that although this journey isn't going to be easy, we must embrace it. This journey is marked by heartache, tenderness, connection, triumphs, resilience, and, most importantly, enhancing the well-being of those we love. It is a journey that I know intimately.

My name is Mary Ann, and just like many of you, I have walked through this emotional and complex path of dementia caregiving. It is no easy task in the slightest, but we have the ability to cope with it. It's a path that will continually test our boundaries of love, compassion, and patience. It will often leave us scared, uncertain, utterly overwhelmed, and even, at

INTRODUCTION

times, painfully alone. On the other hand, the same journey will also be filled with beautiful moments overflowing with connection and love; it is a journey that proves to us just how magnificent the human heart is and how resilient we can be.

I remember my first day when I took on the role of being my beloved grandmother's caregiver. She had recently been diagnosed with Alzheimer's, and I knew immediately that the road ahead would be filled with obstacles for her, myself, and all those who loved her. The initial shock of the recent news was overpowering, and my mind was saturated with questions that seemed to have no answers. "How do I communicate with her? Do I have what it takes to give her the best care and support she deserves? How do I navigate the labyrinthine landscape of dementia care in terms of healthcare, financial, and legal purposes?"

As I took on this newfound path in my life, I discovered that I was not alone and that countless people felt just the way I did. I discovered that there was a profound need for the comprehensive understanding and insights needed for beginners to take on such an important role. Something I would have given the world to possess at the time. Thus, it became my purpose to develop a roadmap for beginner caregivers who were thrust into the world of dementia caregiving without a guiding light to prepare them for what was to come. I wanted to bridge the gap between confusion and confidence, between feeling lost and finding the way forward. This guide is the culmination of that purpose. It's an empathetic companion to prepare you with the understanding, practical skills, and emotional support that you will come to need as you embark on your caregiving journey.

Someone in the world is diagnosed with dementia every three seconds. Currently, approximately 55 million people are

INTRODUCTION

living with dementia globally. There will be 78 million people with dementia worldwide by 2030 and 139 million by 2050. Thus, the need for support, practical guidance, and empathetic solutions for caregivers has never been more prevalent (Alzheimer's Disease International, 2023).

Therefore, join me as we walk this journey together and decode the labyrinth of dementia care. We will explore the many types of dementia and the symptoms we can come to expect; this will form the foundation for your caregiving role. We will expand on this knowledge by exploring effective communication strategies, dismantling the barrier between healthcare professionals and caregivers, discovering practical daily caregiving skills, and arming ourselves with the necessary tools to manage stress and caregiver burnout.

Our journey does not end with the immediate challenges we will face. We will consider and address proactive measures such as building a solid and dependable support network, tackling financial obstacles, and providing a legal roadmap to navigate the complex world of dementia, thus equipping you with what you need to make informed decisions going forward. Lastly, we will cover the grieving process and how we can honor our loved ones' memories upon their passing.

As both a caregiver and an author, I bring forth a wealth of knowledge and personal insights, as I have walked this road before and faced the unique and challenging obstacles you are currently experiencing. I possess the shared understanding that drives me to provide you with the insightful and supportive assistance you require.

While I can't promise you that this will be an easy journey, I can assure you that it will be both fulfilling and rewarding. We need to recognize that we all possess the remarkable capa-

INTRODUCTION

bility to make a great impact in the lives of our loved ones, and I am here to help you channel that inner brilliance and resilience through guidance and support in every step of your journey.

CHAPTER 1
DEMENTIA UNVEILED: TYPES, STAGES, SYMPTOMS, AND PROGRESSION

To fully comprehend the intricate nature of dementia, a neurological disorder that impacts both our cognitive state and our overall quality of life, we must delve into the many aspects and complications of this condition.

Together, we will gradually unravel this complex condition. Dementia is a maze of both mental and emotional challenges that has a deep impact on both the person who is diagnosed with the condition and the others who decide to care for them. We will explore what dementia is, its varying stages, and how it can affect you and your loved one.

DECODING DEMENTIA: MORE THAN JUST MEMORY LOSS

Dementia is a general term used in the medical world to define a wide spectrum of cognitive degeneration and challenges spanning a variety of brain-related conditions. However, contrary to popular belief, dementia is far more than mere memory loss. Unfortunately, this devastating condition impairs not only memory but also decision-making capabilities, the ability to problem-solve, and the ability to perform simple everyday tasks. Dementia causes a lot of stress for everybody involved because it is a form of total cognitive decline and a disease we cannot completely cure. Even though medications are available, they are meant to slow down degeneration rather than to put an end to it entirely.

People who suffer from dementia generally experience varying degrees of memory loss, and as time goes by, the severity of memory loss intensifies. They will struggle to recall recent events, often mix up names and faces, and forget long-term memories as the condition progresses. This can even lead to forgetting family members, lifelong friends, and milestone events in their lives. However, beyond memory, their ability to problem-solve gets greatly diminished, leading to simple everyday tasks becoming increasingly difficult to execute on their own. Simple tasks like dressing themselves, brushing their teeth, and preparing meals become challenging. Disorientation with daily reality and behavior changes are other common symptoms that present themselves as the condition worsens (Dementia Australia, 2014).

The reality is that these symptoms have a severe impact on an individual's quality of life. Thus, we must execute appropriate care to support those diagnosed with dementia, their caregivers, and their families so they have the necessary tools to manage the complexities of this disease. We need to be aware of any warning signs of dementia so that we can detect the disease early on in the process before it progresses drastically, leading to deteriorating symptoms. At the same time, we need to understand that no two people experience dementia the same way (Dementia Australia, 2014).

THE MANY FACES OF DEMENTIA: UNDERSTANDING THE DIFFERENT TYPES

Dementia is an umbrella term encompassing various cognitive impairments, with certain variants being more common than others. It's essential to recognize the diversity within this condition. Thus, it is not a singular condition we can pinpoint right away; however, according to a study conducted in 2020, it was found that the most prevalent of these conditions was undoubtedly Alzheimer's disease. The study found that 60% to 80% of all dementia cases were a result of Alzheimer's. Other relatively common variants of dementia include Vascular Dementia (about 10% of all cases) and Frontotemporal Dementia (about 3% of all cases). Highlighting what type of dementia a person is diagnosed with is crucial to understanding the appropriate care we provide for each patient (Alzheimer's Association, 2023).

There are over 100 different forms of dementia; however, there are five prominent faces of this disease we need to be most vigilant about (Dementia Australia, 2023).

Alzheimer's Disease
This form of dementia is without a doubt the most common form of the disease and one we need to become very familiar with.

Alzheimer's disease is best understood as the accumulation of abnormal proteins festering in the brain. What this essentially means is that the brain's neurons become disrupted, hindering how these neurons communicate with one another. An individual with Alzheimer's disease will experience a decrease in vital chemicals in their brain, which will stop messages from effectively traveling through the brain.

This leads to debilitating symptoms such as:

- Short-term memory loss, including important dates, faces, events, and what they did that day. As the disease progresses, long-term memory also gets affected
- Difficulty in planning, problem-solving, organizing, and thinking logically
- Taking longer to do routine tasks - going to the toilet, eating, getting dressed, etc.
- Language and comprehension difficulties/problems finding the right word/Vagueness in conversation
- Disorientation regarding people, times, and places

It's difficult to pinpoint the exact progression rates of Alzheimer's as different patients deteriorate at different times. It is unique to the patient. However, Alzheimer's is a disease that will eventually lead to a gradual decline in cognitive functioning. In the early stages, individ-uals will face memory difficulties. As the disease progresses to the middle stages, individuals' language, behavior, and judgment will be the next to be affected, and at this stage, more care will be needed. Finally, as this disease reaches its climactic last stages, mobility and independence will be severely impacted, which will most likely result in those diagnosed with dementia needing extensive care. (Dementia Australia, 2022).

Frontotemporal Dementia

The primary difference between Frontotemporal Dementia (FTD) and Alzheimer's disease is that memory often remains unaffected or severely less affected compared to other variants of dementia, particularly in its early stages. The characteristics of Frontotemporal Dementia can be attributed to four impairments: personality, behavior, language, and movement. Essentially, what causes this variant is the fact that there is progressive damage to either or both the frontal or temporal lobes of the brain.

This causes a slew of debilitating symptoms, ranging from:

- loss of language skills, also known as progressive aphasia

- sudden behavior change: appearing selfish or reluctant to adapt to new situations

- loss of empathy and emotional warmth

- loss of interest in hobbies that once interested them,

- avoidance of social gatherings, and lack of motivation

- loss of normal inhibitions exhibiting inappropriate behavior or partaking in embarrassing behavior

- become impulsive and easily distracted

- reasoning, planning, and judgment become clouded

Generally, in the early stages of FTD, the inflicted will suffer from decreased language capabilities (progressive aphasia). Soon after, the disease will progress, and their behavior and personality will start to subtly change and worsen over time. At first, the challenges that they may face include social detachment, emotional blunting, language difficulties, and poor impulse control.

As time goes on, these symptoms will only become more pronounced and can lead to total social isolation and occupational challenges. Finally, as this variant progresses into its late stages, they will suffer from communication difficulties, making it hard to understand others and to express themselves. Some individuals with FTD also suffer from memory issues, executive dysfunction, and difficulty with daily activities; however, these symptoms are not as severe as other dementia variants and are generally rarer symptoms of FTD (Dementia Australia, 2014b).

Vascular Dementia

Vascular dementia is the second-most prevalent variant of dementia and makes up around 10% of all dementia cases. The primary problems that arise from this variant include a lack of reasoning, hindered judgment, poor planning capabilities, disorientation, deteriorating memory, and a shorter attention span. Collectively, these can severely affect an individual's quality of life and ability to socialize or work effectively.

Several catalysts can cause vascular dementia; these include a history of strokes, high blood pressure, high cholesterol, obesity, diabetes, heart disease, blood vessel disease, abnormalities of one's heartbeat, and smoking. Ultimately, vascular dementia is a result of restricted blood flow to the brain, which leads to brain damage.

The restricted flow of blood to the brain can lead to various symptoms, most notably:

- mild to severe memory challenges
- behavioral changes
- deterioration of logical thinking and practical reasoning

- mobility issues

- often, bladder control can be severely impacted.

- deterioration of reasoning and logical thinking capabilities

However, vascular dementia is one of the most challenging forms of dementia to accurately diagnose, as the symptoms for this variant often overlap with multiple other dementia variants. Thus, there is a high probability that those suffering from vascular dementia are also afflicted with Alzheimer's disease and other cognitive illnesses.

Like any other dementia, there is no cure; however, there are a few treatments you can adopt to try to slow down the progression and stabilize vascular dementia. For people who smoke, immediately quitting the habit is one way to stop the symptoms from getting worse; another way is to take Alzheimer's medication (as they are most likely suffering from this too) This will help improve memory, thinking capabilities, and behavior to a certain extent. A healthy diet and adopting a routine exercise schedule will help reduce the chances of suffering from another stroke. Occupational therapy is another option to consider as this can improve mobility and consequently instill a sense of independence.

The rate of progression of vascular dementia is not one-size-fits-all and vastly differs from person to person. However, there is a pattern that can be identified. In the early stages, the individuals will show subtle cognitive changes, such as mild memory challenges, and face difficulty with reasoning and planning. In the mid-stages, cognitive degeneration worsens, leading to memory, language, and behavioral difficulties. In its final stages, the inflicted will suffer from severe cognitive decline and eventual functional deterioration. Essentially, the afflicted will require extra care as their memory, mobility, communication, and independence will be profoundly impacted (Dementia Australia, 2015).

Lewy Body Dementia

Lewy Body is a tricky variant, as Lewy Bodies are present in both Parkinson's disease and dementia. Both Parkinson's and Lewy Body Dementia are incredibly similar to one another, as they both share almost identical symptoms and both viciously attack the brain's cells, making it difficult to accurately diagnose. Essentially, what this means is that inside the brains of people who suffer from Parkinson's and dementia exist microscopic structures known as Lewy bodies. These structures consist of a protein known as alpha-synuclein that, for reasons the medical world is still unclear, gets tangled up. This results in the gradual loss of brain cells, which ultimately leads to decreased mobility, hindered thinking, and behavioral alterations.

Lewy Body disease is a highly complex cognitive ailment that technically has three overlapping disorders. One of these disorders is Parkinson's disease, which is typically categorized as a cognitive disorder that harshly impacts a person's movement and is often attributed to severe muscle stiffness and muscle tremors. The Second disorder is a continuation of the first and is known as Parkinson's Disease Dementia. This occurs when typical dementia symptoms begin to present themselves in addition to the symptoms of Parkinson's Disease. This generally occurs at least a year after being diagnosed with Parkinson's, and the progression to dementia is relatively slow-acting. The final overlapping disorder is known as Lewy Bodies Dementia and will typically present itself in patients at least a year before any mobility issues. However, it is important to note that visual hallucinations may be experienced with this variant of dementia, and if that is the case, it's important to seek immediate medical expertise.

There are several early warning signs to watch out for that could aid in the early detection of Lewy Body disease, so be on the lookout for:

- poor sense of smell or a complete loss of scent
- lack of interest or enthusiasm, particularly in what usually brings the person joy
- increased anxiety and potentially an onslaught of depression
- constipation and urinary incontinence
- fainting
- abnormal drowsiness and fatigue
- in rare cases, people may suffer from delusions and halluci-nations

Due to Lewy Body disease having so many overlapping conditions, symptoms will largely depend on what area of the brain has been affected; this will also determine the progression of the disease (Dementia Australia, 2014c).

STAGES OF DEMENTIA: THE JOURNEY FROM EARLY TO LATE STAGE

When a person is diagnosed with dementia, particularly Alzheimer's disease, they are typically given a life expectancy of four to eight years; however, many people with this dreaded disease have gone on to live for over 20 years after their initial diagnosis. It drastically varies from person to person. However, dementia is not a stagnant disease; it gets progressively worse as time marches on(Alzheimer's Association, 2022).

Cognitive-related changes typically begin manifesting years before the symptoms truly present themselves. When describing dementia's cycle of progression, three stages are categorized as mild (early stage), moderate (mid-stage), and severe (late stage). Remember, not everybody will progress through these stages at the same rate, as dementia comes with varying degrees of manifestation and intensity in different people (Alzheimer's Association, 2022).

Early Stages of Dementia

In this stage, many people will still be able to maintain a competent level of independence; however, some challenges they may face in these early stages include:

• difficulty in finding the right words, recalling names (especially when meeting new people), and sometimes faces

• start to struggle to a degree in social and workplace settings

• forget content they have recently read or seen

• misplace important items like their phone, wallet, or keys

• difficulty with organizing or planning

• some individuals may experience issues with their vision or balance, making it difficult to read or drive

The reality is that these symptoms can be debilitating, but they are not glaringly obvious to the naked eye. Oftentimes, friends, family, colleagues, and people who interact with the afflicted every day will fail to notice these symptoms and changes in cognitive behavior (Alzheimer's Association, 2022).

That being said, there are several other warning signs beyond the challenges I have mentioned that we should be made aware of. Understanding these additional warning signs helps us detect dementia early and plan before it progresses more aggressively. These signs are as follows:

1. Forgetting recently learned information: This includes forgetting important dates or events, relying on memory aids (notes and phone notifications), relying on people close to them to remember details they could normally recall on their own, or asking the same questions over and over.

2. Finding it difficult to solve problems: Often, people who suffer from dementia, even in the early stages, will find it difficult to think logically and follow a plan. This could be something like struggling to follow a familiar recipe, taking far longer to complete a task that would generally take seconds to complete, or finding it difficult to keep track of their monthly bills when this was never an issue before.

3. Difficulty with accomplishing simple routine tasks: This could be getting lost while driving, even if it is a route they take home every day. Getting confused when organizing a grocery list or failing to remember the rules of their favorite card game even though they have been playing it with their friends for years

4. Becoming disoriented with both time and place: At times, individuals suffering from dementia will not understand why something isn't happening immediately or will become confused about how they got to a particular place. At times, they may not know what that place is, even if they have been there multiple times.

5. Decreased or poor judgment: Some of the telling signs of this could be neglecting their hygiene or being reckless with their finances

6. They may remove themselves from social activities: This is often because they struggle to hold a conversation, lose enthu-siasm for the hobbies that once brought them joy, or feel embar-rassed as they notice they are becoming increasingly forgetful

7. You may notice some behavioral changes in them: During this stage, individuals may experience confusion, suspicion, depression, fear, or anxiety. They might become easily upset in familiar settings, with friends, or when they're outside their comfort zone.

Remember, these are just warning signs we need to be alert to; it does not necessarily mean people with dementia will show all these signs, some may only show a few of them (Alzheimer's Association, 2019).

Middle Stages of Dementia

In the middle stages of dementia, symptoms become more aggressive. Individuals will experience more severe memory challenges, difficulty expressing themselves, confuse their words more regularly, struggle with routine tasks, and behave in uncharacteristic ways. They may also become more irritable, frustrated, and angry, often acting irrationally.

This is usually the longest stage of dementia and can last for several years. In these middle stages, there is a high probability that the afflicted will need a greater level of care.

Common symptoms during this stage include:

• forgetting important events, in addition to their personal history

- inability to recall personal information like address, phone number, part of their childhood or young adulthood, or even where they attended school

- greater confusion regarding place and time

- difficulty in selecting appropriate clothing for a specific occasion or season

- difficulty controlling their bladder and bowel

- sleeping patterns get altered; for example, they may sleep during the day but become restless at night

- increased tendency to get lost or wander around

- changes in personality and behavior, such as skepticism delusions, or repetitive actions

In this stage, your loved one can still participate in daily activities; however, they will most likely need assistance. As a caregiver, it is important to figure out what your loved one can still do on their own or find solutions to simplify tasks for them. As dementia progresses and the symptoms worsen, caregivers may want to consider respite care or an adult day center so they can have a temporary break from caregiving while still having the peace of mind that those they love are still getting the quality care they need in a safe environment (Alzheimer's Association, 2022).

Late Stages of Dementia

In the final stage of dementia, symptoms become severe, and your loved ones will require extensive care. Those living with the late stages of dementia will struggle more profusely with communication, worsening memory, movement challenges, and notable personality changes. Individuals in the late stages of dementia find it increasingly difficult to respond to their environment.

In these late stages, the afflicted may:

- require 24/7 personal care
- become unaware of recent experiences and their surroundings
- experience challenges with their physical capabilities, such as walking, sitting, and even swallowing
- become more susceptible to infections, particularly pneumonia.
- have difficulty communicating

In these late stages of dementia, individuals may find it difficult to initiate engagement with those around them; however, they can still benefit from appropriate alternative interactions such as calming music or receiving comfort from gentle physical touch. In these severe stages, caregivers may opt to explore support services such as hospices, which are designed to provide individuals with comfort and dignity in the final stages of life. Hospices provide invaluable assistance to both those suffering from dementia as well as to families caring for their loved ones (Alzheimer's Association, 2022).

THE PROGRESSION PUZZLE: UNDERSTANDING DEMENTIA'S IMPACT OVER TIME

By understanding the different stages of dementia, you are equipped with the knowledge you will need to effectively provide care, emotional support, therapies, and timely interventions to address the specific cognitive, emotional, and functional challenges your loved ones are dealing with at any given point during their dementia journey.

As dementia progresses, more intensive caregiving is necessary as your loved ones' mental and physical capabilities increasingly deteriorate. According to a World Health Organization report, caregivers have to comprehend this process because it has the potential to have a detrimental impact on their own physical and mental health, often referred to as caregiver burnout (World Health Organization, 2023). This highlights the paramount importance of placing a high value on caregiver health in the face of the severe challenges brought on as dementia evolves through its stages.

CHAPTER 2
DECODING MEDICAL JARGON: BRIDGING THE GAP BETWEEN CAREGIVERS AND HEALTHCARE PROVIDERS

Understanding the intricacies of medical jargon and mastering the art of effective communication with healthcare providers is a crucial skill for a caregiver's journey.

Together, we will explore the insights that medical terminology holds. We will be demystifying complex terms and medical reports, in addition to learning how to advocate on behalf of our loved ones and ensure that their needs are met appropriately.

Acquiring this insight enables caregivers to navigate the medical sector with confidence. We will learn effective techniques to bridge the communication gap between healthcare professionals and caregivers, enabling open, informed, and cooperative dialogue. These skills will ultimately improve the standard of care for our loved ones and gives us the peace of mind from understanding their care plan.

DECODING MEDICAL JARGON: BRIDGING THE GAP
BETWEEN CAREGIVERS AND HEALTHCARE PROVIDERS

BREAKING DOWN MEDICAL TERMINOLOGY: UNDERSTANDING THE BASICS

Navigating the world of medical jargon can be an overwhelming experience. Understanding the meaning of these complex terms, abbreviations, and technical phrases can often leave us feeling baffled and even anxious. To make this journey more manageable, you can find a comprehensive glossary of the medical terms and abbreviations you will need at the end of this book. If you encounter terms like "sundowning", "aphasia", "MRI," or any other confusing medical terms, don't hesitate to turn to the glossary for clarity and a deeper understanding.

EMPOWERING CAREGIVERS: ASKING THE RIGHT QUESTIONS OF HEALTHCARE PROVIDERS

When caregivers understand the appropriate questions to ask their loved one's healthcare professionals, it empowers them to obtain the exact information and tools they require to support those they care for.

Some questions you may want to consider asking include:

"What stage of dementia is my loved one in?"

This provides caregivers with crucial insights regarding care treatments, how to communicate, legal and financial matters, preparing themselves emotionally, and tailoring care to improve their loved one's quality of life.

"What changes should I expect in their behavior as the disease progresses?"

Setting expectations in advance might help you get ready for your loved one's future needs. Whether that means modifying your house for the care of a loved one, exploring memory care services before you truly need them, or other adaptive measures will depend on how your loved one's dementia progresses.

"As a caregiver, what are the most pressing matters I need to be made aware of about my loved one's care?"

This question ensures that you and the medical professional are on the same page and agree on the expected course of action.

"What are the latest treatments available, and which treatment plan do you suggest will be most effective?"

This is a question that you are going to want to ask throughout your loved one's care journey with their doctor. This is because dementia treatment is forever evolving, and treatments that were used at the beginning of a diagnosis may not be as effective as the new treatment plans available now.

"How can I make my home safer for my loved one?"

Dementia patients often suffer from delirium and aimless wandering, posing safety risks to themselves. Therefore, it is best to find out from healthcare professionals what the best course of action is to manage the home environment for the well-being and safety of your loved one.

"Which warning signs should I watch out for during visits, and what actions justify an emergency response?"

While dementia is a horrid disease and we should always pay attention to our loved one's behavior changes as a result of dementia, we need to remember that not all changes warrant panic or an emergency response. To help put your mind at ease, it is always wise to ask your doctor about what behavior changes are anticipated versus ones that should raise concerns.

"Are there any side effects to this medication, and what is the dose and frequency of the medication?" (only ask if medication is prescribed.)

While most medications will stipulate both the side effects and dosage printed on the label of the packaging, it is always best to discuss them with your doctor first in case you have further questions. This could potentially save you from stress later on.

"How will this affect the overall quality of life for my loved one, and could these treatments/procedures lead to additional problems?" (Only if the doctor suggests running major diagnostic tests or treatment.)

Be certain that you completely understand the recommended course of action and how it will impact your loved one's outcome and quality of life.

"What are the next steps?"

Having an open and frank discussion with your loved one's doctor about the eventualities that will arise will alleviate some of the stress of future decisions. Discuss future decisions long before your loved one needs any of these, such as assisted living, nursing homes, adult day care services, palliative care, and hospice (Bristal, 2021).

DEVELOPING A RAPPORT WITH YOUR DOCTOR

Establishing a good rapport with your neurologist is critical for smoother communication. By fostering this relationship, you will create an environment where the exchange of vital information becomes seamless and more effective. This will ultimately lead to more effective care, as it allows your neurologist to become better acquainted with your loved one's unique needs.

To build this report, it is wise to regularly update your doctor about any noticeable changes in your loved one's behavior or overall health. This acquired knowledge can prove extremely helpful for doctors. As a result of this constant flow of communication, healthcare providers are empowered to tailor their approach when treating your loved one, which ensures that treatment will remain responsive and aligned to the evolving state of dementia.

Make sure you are consistently scheduling appointments with your healthcare professional and are proactively seeking advice from them. This will help foster a more comprehensive care plan, resulting in both short-term and long-term strategies being developed for managing your loved one's dementia care.

Remember that open, honest, and clear communication with your neurologist is essential.

Don't be afraid to ask any follow-up questions or seek clarification on certain aspects of the treatment you may not fully understand. By being well-informed, you are equipping yourself with all the tools you need to make proper decisions and ensure that your loved one is getting the best possible care available. This collaborative partnership between caregiver and doctor is essential to enhancing the quality of life of those you care for through their journey with dementia.

MAKING THE MOST OF MEDICAL REPORTS: UNDERSTANDING AND UTILIZING THE INFORMATION

To many, medical reports may just be seen as complex and intricate documents flooded with complicated data and medical jargon that is impossible understand; however, if you can grasp the basics and approach them with understanding and insight, these documents become a goldmine filled with rich information. These reports often hold the secrets crucial for doctors and even caregivers to evaluate the state of a patient's cognitive health and provide a metric to track the progression of dementia. When it comes to medical reports and tests, we can categorize them into three groups: lab test results, imaging scans, and doctor's notes.

Lab Test Results

These results can be used to gather a comprehensive look into a patient's cognitive and psychological well-being. They are incredibly useful to extract vital information about a patient's blood chemistry, organ function, and any other potential abnormalities in the body. If the results come back with either elevated or diminished values compared to what is considered normal, it could signal a multitude of underlying conditions and act as a guiding light for doctors to effectively diagnose and treat various ailments. These tests can assist doctors in ruling out any other potential causes of cognitive degeneration. Common lab tests include blood tests, genetic tests, and cerebrospinal fluid analysis.

The most common of these tests would be a blood test. They are conducted to rule out other potential causes of cognitive degeneration, such as vitamin deficiency, thyroid abnormalities, or a metabolic disorder; all of these could mimic the symptoms that are present in dementia.

Another test doctors use to diagnose dementia is known as genetic testing. This would be employed if there is a family history of dementia, as certain genes like APOE-e04 can be carried over in offspring and run the risk of developing into specific dementia types, particularly Alzheimer's. However, this is extremely rare and The Alzheimer's Association advises against conducting routine genetic testing for Alzheimer's disease risk without first ensuring that an individual has received adequate counseling and comprehends the essential information required to make an informed decision (Alzheimer's Association, 2019a).

Additionally, a medical exam known as cerebrospinal fluid analysis could be used. This test is executed through a lumbar puncture to detect abnormal proteins linked to specific dementias, like Alzheimer's.

Imaging Scans

There are three primary types of imaging scans, which include a computed tomography (CT) scan, a magnetic resonance imaging (MRI) scan, or a positron emission tomography (PET) scan. A CT scan is used to quickly detect any structural issues in the brain; an MRI scan is similar to a CT scan but offers a more detailed scan of the brain to gain a clearer picture of what's going on; and a PET scan is used to assess the brain's metabolism and beta-amyloid plaques (a clump of proteins on the brain). In a nutshell, all these scans are employed to provide the medical team with detailed images of the internal structures of the brain. Ultimately, this will help the doctors identify any structural abnormalities, including tumors, strokes, brain atrophy, and dementia. These are powerful scans and not only will they be able to confirm the presence of dementia conditions, but will also be able to determine the extent of its progression (Dementia Australia, 2014d).

Doctor's Notes

These notes essentially act as the narrative thread that weaves together a full picture of the patient's medical history and journey. These notes will generally contain a wealth of information, including their neurological exams, cognitive assessments, motor skills results, the speed of their reflexes, and the extent of their coordination. Any abnormalities within these results can indicate the severity and type of dementia your loved one may be afflicted with. They offer an invaluable understanding of the complexities and intricate nature of dementia and help healthcare professionals personalize their treatment plan to meet the unique needs of your loved one.

ADVOCATING FOR YOUR LOVED ONE: ENSURING THEIR NEEDS ARE MET

When you become a caregiver, your role extends beyond looking after their needs; you become their biggest supporter, especially when medical matters are concerned, to ensure they are receiving the best care possible. The role of being their trusted advocate extends to expressing their unique preferences, concerns, and essential needs to their doctors. Ultimately, you are ensuring that they receive the dedicated and tailored care they deserve. This could involve seeking a second opinion, researching treatment options, or pushing for additional care services. For instance, if you feel your loved one's current treatment plan is not effective, don't hesitate to discuss other options with the healthcare provider.

Advocacy can present itself in many forms. One of the most prominent ways it manifests itself is by effectively communicating your loved one's wishes to their team of doctors. For instance, if your loved one does not feel entirely comfortable with a particular medical procedure, then it becomes your duty as their caregiver to relay this communication to their doctor. Essentially, your voice acts as the bridge between the patient and the doctor. You are ensuring that your loved one's feelings and desires are both understood and respected by their team of medical professionals.

The truth is, as caregivers, we need to be proactive with our advocacy. We need to recognize that this is not an option but a necessity. By taking the initiative and being proactive, we can significantly impact the treatment plan, which will positively affect both us and our loved one. Don't be afraid to voice your concerns and ask the doctor relevant questions. We need to be both vigilant and assertive in our role as advocates. This will help prevent oversights, misunderstandings, or undergoing treatments beyond your loved one's wishes. Being vigilant is also pivotal in nurturing a collaborative relationship with your loved one's doctors, which will improve the overall quality of care they receive.

At its core, when you adopt the role of an advocate, you become the embodiment of both love and dedication. Being your loved one's steadfast voice allows you to give them the confidence they need to navigate the complex environment of medicine, guaranteeing their desires are considered and respected throughout their journey with dementia.

CHAPTER 3
GRASPING THE BASICS: UNDERSTANDING MEDICAL TREATMENTS FOR DEMENTIA

Dementia is a complex disease that brings many challenges and uncertainties. We might feel puzzled and overwhelmed as we cope with our loved one's condition. . Thus, it is paramount as caregivers that we fully understand the multitude of both medical and non-medical interventions available to our loved ones. Together, we will seek to identify the types of interventions available, with the ultimate goal of choosing the proper ones to help in effectively managing our loved one's dementia symptoms.

As we highlight each of these interventions, you will become better equipped to have empowered and informed discussions with medical providers. Enabling you to make better decisions for the benefit of yourself and your loved one. This chapter is designed to arm you with the resources needed to navigate the intricacies of dementia treatments with confidence and understanding throughout your loved one's dementia journey.

GRASPING THE BASICS: UNDERSTANDING MEDICAL TREATMENTS FOR DEMENTIA

It is important to note that while medication cannot cure dementia, it is still crucial in managing, stabilizing, and slowing down the progression of dementia symptoms. These medications aim to improve the quality of life of individuals diagnosed with dementia, in addition to providing relief from behavioral and cognitive symptoms. Two primary drug classes are used to manage dementia symptoms: cholinesterase inhibitors and memantine.

Dementia medications are approved by doctors at specific stages: early, middle, and late stages, and will be administered based on the patient's cognitive assessment results. However, they will not be administered if it is found a patient is diagnosed with mild cognitive impairment (MCI); this is the transition stage between age-related cognitive decline and dementia-related cognitive degeneration. These medications mentioned have shown limited benefit in MCI patients or any preventative measures in preventing MCI from progressing into dementia.

Cholinesterase Inhibitors

These drugs work by boosting levels of a chemical messenger involved in memory and judgment. This drug class is commonly used to treat mild to moderate Alzheimer's disease. There is a chemical in the brain known as acetylcholine that decreases in individuals who suffer from dementia. When this chemical decreases, both alertness and memory become impaired. Thus, this drug is administered to help stop acetylcholine from breaking down; however, while cholinesterase is effective in managing both the decline of memory and alertness, it cannot reverse or completely stop the effects of dementia.

There are a couple of common side effects of cholinesterase inhibitors that one should be aware of. These include (American Family Physician, 2018):

- nausea
- vomiting
- diarrhea
- decreased appetite
- muscle cramps
- fatigue
- insomnia
- dizziness
- headaches
- indigestion

The risk of suffering from these common side effects can be decreased with a low dose, gradually increasing it, and taking the medication after eating. It is not wise for individuals with cardiac arrhythmias (heart rhythm issues) to take this medication.

Within the cholinesterase inhibitor drug class, there are three commonly prescribed medications:

• Donepezil: This medication can be used to treat all stages of dementia and should be taken once a day.

• Galantamine: This is generally used to treat moderate or mid-stage dementia and should be taken once a day.

GRASPING THE BASICS: UNDERSTANDING MEDICAL TREATMENTS FOR DEMENTIA

Additionally, this medication can be taken twice a day as an extended-release capsule.

• Rivastigmine: Typically used to treat early or mid-stage dementia and is taken as a pill or a skin patch. In some cases, doctors will administer this drug to treat late stages of dementia (Mayo Clinic, 2019a)

Memantine

Memantine, also known as Namenda, is approved by the Food and Drug Administration (FDA) to treat individuals who are diagnosed with mid-stage and late-stage dementia. Essentially, what this drug class does is regulate glutamate, a crucial brain chemical that facilitates memory and learning.

Memantine can come in both syrup and pill form and has some common side effects you should be aware of (Mayo Clinic, 2019):

• dizziness

• headache

• confusion

• agitation or nervousness

• weight gain

• bloating of the face, arms, hands, lower legs, or feet

• tingling in hands and feet

• slower or faster heartbeat

Regular check-ups are essential for your loved one's doctors to assess medication response and effectiveness. This helps them decide if any adjustments are necessary or if the medication can remain unchanged.

BEYOND PILLS: NON-MEDICAL INTERVENTIONS FOR DEMENTIA

Managing dementia goes beyond pharmaceutical treatment and often encompasses a more holistic lifestyle approach. By fostering a more holistic lifestyle, you will enhance your loved one's overall well-being and quality of life. These approaches highlight that dementia is far more complex than what the general public believes and affects more than just one cognitive function; in fact, it impacts their emotional, physical, and social well-being. We will uncover in depth some holistic approaches to add to your loved one's overall treatment plan.

A Balanced Diet

There is one diet that all individuals diagnosed with dementia should be eating, and that is the MIND diet (Mediterranean-DASH Intervention for Neurodegenerative Delay). The MIND diet is made up of two diets, known as the Mediterranean diet and the Dash diet.

The Mediterranean diet is made up of foods that, when combined, provide antioxidants, anti-inflammatory compounds, and nutrients that, according to research from Harvard Medical School, lower rates of dementia. The diet consists of fruits, vegetables, whole grains, lean protein sources, and healthy fats like olive oil.

The second diet that makes up the MIND diet is the DASH (Dietary Approaches to Stop Hypertension) diet. This diet is recommended for people who want to prevent high blood pressure and reduce the risk of strokes and heart disease, which is a primary factor in vascular dementia. This diet consists of fruits, vegetables, whole grains, and lean meats.

Nutrition is a crucial aspect of managing dementia, and while it may not cure the disease, it will help manage symptoms and improve your loved one's overall quality of life (Harvard University, 2022).

Physical Exercise

Physical exercise is a fantastic approach to not only help manage dementia systems and improve the well-being of those living with the disease, but it is also very effective in helping reduce the risk of developing dementia later in life. Countless studies have shown that there is a direct link between cognitive health and physical activity.

There are some incredible exercises out there that individuals living with dementia can engage in daily to enhance their blood flow to the brain, such as walking, light jogging, swimming, gentle yoga, Tai Chi, and even gardening. The increased blood flow to the brain can stimulate the growth and survival of brain cells, which could slow down and manage cognitive decline. Additionally, if your loved one can, undergoing light strength and resistance training can help build muscle strength, improve flexibility, and support metabolic health, thus aiding in the slower progression of mobility impairment brought on by dementia variants.

Maintaining a routine of exercise is crucial for individuals who already have dementia. It may assist in preventing muscle deterioration, mobility problems, and other ailments brought on by inactivity. Your loved ones should incorporate a regular exercise schedule in the early stages of dementia, as this can provide monumental benefits as the disease progresses (Dementia Australia, 2015b).

Incorporating physical activity into daily routines can make these beneficial habits easier to maintain. Make use of these tips and tricks to help get your loved ones physically active and maintain both their mobility and strength:

- **Play music while exercising:** Not only will this make exer-cise more enjoyable for your loved one, but it has also been found that people living with dementia respond positively to music. If at all possible, incorporate dancing along to the music, as this is a highly effective way to get the blood pumping and maintain connections with your loved one, in addition to being enjoyable for them.

- **Go on walks together:** This will help you maintain connec-tions and motivate your loved ones. Don't forget that care-givers need exercise too!

- **Be realistic:** Identify what you honestly believe they can achieve in one exercise session; don't overdo it. It may be wise to incorporate several "mini-workouts" that are short and easily manageable.

- **Wear the right clothing:** Make sure your loved one is wearing comfortable clothing that is not too big or too small for them, and make sure their shoes are appropriate for exer-cising to avoid blisters.

- **Make use of YouTube, your local TV guide, or programs:** There are plenty of free videos and programs designed for elderly workouts to give you ideas about which exercises you could include in your loved ones' workouts.

Naturally, as symptoms of cognitive degeneration and mobility impairments become more severe as dementia progresses, exercising becomes increasingly more challeng-ing. However, even in these later stages, individuals with dementia may still be able to:

- Do simple tasks around the home with assistance, such as sweeping and dusting.

- Use a stationary bike.

- Exercise with rubber bands, exercise balls or balloons. They could be used to help stretch or to throw back and forth with their caregiver.

- Make use of stretching bands to engage in gentle stretching exercises

- Lift light weights (2kg or lighter) or household items such as soup cans.

(National Institute of Aging, 2017)

However, you should first check with their doctors before starting an exercise program to make sure which exercises are appropriate.

Mental Stimulation

Keeping your mind occupied and active is equally important. Just a few examples of activities that are likely to stimulate the mind include puzzles, reading, and listening to music. Music has a remarkable capacity to evoke emotions, awaken memories, and sharpen thoughts. It gives those who might have difficulty expressing their emotions verbally an effective alternative.

Puzzles and reading are also effective mental activities, as they require a lot of focus and mental fortitude to engage in these activities, thus stimulating the brain's mental capacity (Berg-Weger & Stewart, 2017).

Reminiscence Therapy
This is a form of non-pharmaceutical therapy that helps harness the power of your loved one's memory to improve their overall well-being. It is executed by using tangible items as memory aids, such as childhood mementos, cherished items, photos from years past, films they adore, and music. By using these reminiscent memory aids, we can tap into a reservoir of cherished memories that individuals who suffer from dementia often hold onto, as they are linked to their sense of self. These memories exist as childhood memories, inseparable relationships, personal achievements, and life milestones.

It is important to engage in guided discussions with your loved ones to help them share their past with you, offering them an opportunity for a therapeutic outlet to emotionally express themselves without overbearing their cognitive func-tions. Reminiscence therapy has shown to be empathetic and supportive, whether it is employed in group settings, to develop a sense of community via shared memories, or for individual-focused life evaluations.

This kind of therapy enriches the lives of those you care for and helps them hold on to their identity amid memory impairment. In essence, this form of therapy helps manage their cognitive and depressive symptoms (Berg-Weger & Stewart, 2017).

Validation Therapy
This approach is designed to improve our communication with our loved ones diagnosed with early to middle stages of dementia. The ultimate aim of this approach is to both recog-nize and affirm the emotions and self-identity of our loved ones. It is based on the premise that confusion serves as a

coping mechanism for those living with dementia to manage stress, overcome boredom, reduce loneliness, or escape from their reality.

As caregivers, we wear many hats. One of those hats is the facilitator. This means we do not try to dispel or correct our loved one's confusion but rather acknowledge and validate their feelings and emotions as truth, even if they are not. It might sound strange, but it helps reduce stress, improve feelings of contentment, and reduce behavioral changes. In a nutshell, this approach prioritizes validating an individual's emotions and feelings during times of disorientation rather than trying to instill factual accuracy (Berg-Weger & Stewart, 2017).

Pet Therapy

We all love pets. Pets are extremely calming for individuals with dementia and can help them communicate. The act of caring for a pet offers individuals with dementia valuable support, espe-cially for those who struggle to communicate effectively or maintain a conversation. Pet therapy, or animal-assisted inter-ventions, have been found to enhance self-esteem and confi-dence in individuals with dementia. Pet therapy can enhance the overall quality of life and foster a sense of independence for our loved ones living with dementia (Alzheimer's Society, 2020).

Aroma Therapy

Dementia patients have shown significant benefits from aromatherapy. This therapy is designed to activate the olfactory receptors, which are proteins that are essential to the sense of smell as they bind aroma molecules together. Once these are activated, they stimulate the part of the brain that is responsible for alleviating both anxiety and depressive symptoms.

A variety of essential oils have been shown to enhance memory and cognitive performance for those living with dementia. Two of the most challenging dementia symptoms to address are agitation and aggression. Studies have demonstrated the calming effects of some essential oils, most notably lavender, bergamot, and lemon balm, which have been known to reduce the severity of agitation, aggression, and other psychotic symptoms in people diagnosed with dementia (Betsaida, 2018).

THE ROLE OF REGULAR MEDICAL CHECKUPS

Schedule continuous check-ups with your loved one's neurologist and any other member of the medical team who is caring for them, which is essential for ensuring comprehensive care and management of symptoms throughout their dementia journey. Every check-up provides you and the doctors with an opportunity to closely monitor the progression of dementia and evaluate or alter the treatment plan based on its effectiveness.

Through regular checkups and assessments, changes in cognitive ability, mood, behavior, and physical health can be quickly identified, either signaling to healthcare professionals that the treatment plan is working or that there may need to be adjustments to the current treatment strategy. Due to dementia being a progressive disease by nature, we need to be proactive so that we do not allow dementia to rapidly advance without proper intervention beforehand.

Beyond monitoring the effectiveness or the need to change a treatment plan, these regular checkups provide the caregiver with an essential platform to voice their concerns, ask questions, and seek further guidance.

GRASPING THE BASICS: UNDERSTANDING MEDICAL TREATMENTS FOR DEMENTIA

Caregivers generally notice minor alterations in the behavior and health of their loved ones, which may not necessarily be immediately noticeable to healthcare professionals as they are not with the patient regularly. Often, caregivers will find that there is a pattern of increased delirium or agitation in the later hours of the afternoon and at night; this is commonly known as "sundowning", Discussing this with their doctor during one of their check-ups can lead to valuable insights for both yourself and the doctor. Often, in this case, a neurologist will simply recommend altering the timing of medication administration or help formulate a calming evening routine to address your loved one's sundowning habits.

Collaboration and efficient interaction between the patient, caregiver, and medical team are crucial to ensuring effective and holistic management of dementia. Regular checkups are crucial in ensuring this collaborative partnership of care, as they facilitate continual and open dialogue. Prioritizing these meetings with neurologists and other doctors is vital to improving the quality of life of your loved one and forms the foundation for strategizing a thorough and personalized care plan tailored to their unique needs.

CHAPTER 4
FINDING THE RIGHT WORDS: SUCCESSFUL COMMUNICATION WITH DEMENTIA PATIENTS

As caregivers, our job is not easy by any means; however, few, if any, challenges are as pervasive and poignant as the ongoing barrier between our loved ones and ourselves as we journey through the complexities of dementia. Due to the nature of this condition, our loved ones are unable to communicate as they had in the past, which makes it challenging for us to understand their needs and respond accordingly.

This pain point is extremely prevalent and mutually experienced by caregivers from around the globe, which is why we will dive deep into the heart of these communication barriers and highlight the profound importance of connection and understanding throughout the dementia care journey. The primary goal of this chapter is to equip you with the tools you need to engage in effective and empathetic communication that is aligned with the unique needs of those you care deeply for.

THE ART OF PATIENCE: SLOWING DOWN TO CONNECT

As a caregiver caring for our loved one, it is paramount that we are being proactive and that we are the ones initiating communication interactions and conversations. As dementia progresses into its later stages, your loved one will initiate fewer and fewer social interactions by themselves.

Taking that initiative and creating conversation is essential for maintaining a strong connection with your loved one; this engagement does not go unnoticed. One of our many roles as caregivers is establishing a communicative environment that provides our loved ones with a sense of security and connection, which in turn will help them feel heard and valued despite their difficulty initiating conversations with others on their own (NHS, 2023).

To make this process easier for both you and the one you care for, here are several strategies you can implement for verbal communication:

Speak Clearly and Slowly

Whenever you engage in conversation with a person who has dementia, be mindful of your pronunciation and the pace at which you speak. Use short sentences. This will help them process the information at their own pace, reducing confusion.

Give Them Time to Both Process Information and Respond

When communicating with your loved one, patience is essential. Don't get frustrated; they are not ignoring you; they are processing information. People with dementia take far longer to process information than those who do not have the disease. Keep this in mind, and avoid rushing them, as it will only cause unnecessary stress

Try to get them to Socialize With Others

Whenever possible, try to find opportunities for them to get involved and participate in social events or conversations with other people other than you. Social engagement is a superb way to make them feel like they belong and can be highly beneficial for their psychological health.

Let Them Have a voice; Try Not to Speak on Behalf of Them All the Time

If possible, whenever you can see they are managing to hold a conversation on their own, even if they stumble here and there, let them be in charge of the interaction. Whenever there are any discussions about your loved one's welfare and health and they can advocate and speak for themselves regarding the matter, let them. Always avoid patronizing or ridiculing their expressions. It may seem like they are not aware of what's going on, but they are aware of more than we think.

Acknowledge and Encourage

Even if their responses are completely out of context, not factual, and do not directly answer your question, just acknowledge what they said and let them know that they have been heard. This is an example of active listening and encourages your loved one to participate in further conversation later on. For example, if you ask, "How's your weekend going, Gran?" and she replies, "Oh, it's a lovely day today," just acknowledge what she said so she feels heard and respected.

Don't Over-Complicate, Offer Simple Choices

Make decision-making easier and less overwhelming for them by presenting them with simple, straightforward choices rather than a complex array of alternatives. For example, ask them, "Mom, do you want chicken or beef for dinner?" Do not ask something like "Mom, we're getting takeout; do you want chicken, Italian, fish, beef, stew, a roast, sushi, burgers, pie, or Mexican?" Try to keep choices down to two, and make three choices your maximum.

Adapt the Conversation

Be adaptable in the way you communicate. Ask questions again if required, keeping in mind that they might find it difficult to respond as they once did. For instance, you ask, "Gramma, did you play cards today?" and she replies, "Tea with Barb and Marge was lovely, dear, thanks for asking." Play along and just adapt as the conversation goes. You could respond by saying, "Oh, how are Barb and Marge doing? I haven't seen them in ages."

Be Prepared for Repetitive Questions, Be Kind, and Don't Lose Your Cool

One thing that you will certainly experience as a dementia caregiver is tons of repetitive questions. Here's what you do: First, remember that they are not doing this intentionally; their memory loss makes them forget what they've asked before. Secondly, approach these questions with kindness and empathy. If you feel they are getting stuck in a loop, you can try and gently distract them with another topic; this can often be quite helpful (NHS, 2023).

NON-VERBAL COMMUNICATION: BEYOND WORDS

Speaking is only one aspect of communication. You can communicate meaning or help convey a message via gestures, movement, and facial expressions. Studies have found that non-verbal communication makes up approximately 55% of all our communication efforts (The University of Texas, 2020).

This statistic carries paramount importance when communicating with someone who has dementia because they with initiating and understanding verbal communication. Thus, non-verbal signals like body language, hand gestures, facial expressions, and the tone of our voice become essential cues to aid in communication with our loved ones in the absence of fluid verbal conversations (NHS, 2023).

To help simplify the process of non-verbal communication, there are a few strategies you can adopt to make communication efforts smoother:

Maintain Eye Contact and Smile

Maintaining eye contact conveys interest, engagement, and attentiveness and is a superb way to let your loved ones know that they are being heard and respected. Eye contact signals that you are present at the moment and are fully attentive to their needs. While you maintain eye contact, don't forget to put on a warm smile, as this expresses both affection and reassurance, which will ultimately create an environment where your loved ones will feel comfortable during social interactions. The more comfortable they feel, the more willing they will be to contribute to a conversation.

Physical Touch

Gentle physical touch is an effective strategy to establish a connection with your loved ones while conveying a non-verbal message of care. This could be a reassuring pat on their arm, holding their hand while you converse, or engaging in a warm hug. This technique is especially useful when the individual you are caring for finds it difficult to adequately express their emotions verbally. However, you should always be mindful and respectful of your loved ones' personal boundaries and comfort levels. Some people might not want as much physical contact as others

Adopt a Positive Tone

Although many people may not think of the tone of their voice as a kind of non-verbal communication, it is a crucial component. Your tone is essential to setting the emotional atmosphere of a conversation. Try to speak in a warm, soft, positive, and friendly tone whenever possible to create a reas-suring and welcoming environment for your loved ones. Tone can greatly reduce confusion and tension, in addition to encouraging a pleasant conversation.

Keep a Respectable Distance

To avoid intimidating individuals with dementia, it is wise to keep a respectable distance between you and your loved ones during conversations if you find they are becoming agitated. Another tip is to be at eye level with them, especially when you are sitting, as this can further foster a sense of comfort and make them feel less overwhelmed. This creates a psychological sense of equality, in addition to reassuring them that they are not being talked down to.

Engage in Active Listening

It is important to actively motivate your loved ones to express themselves in the manner of their choosing. Acknowledge that certain individuals may become frustrated or overwhelmed in challenging social environments. Because they frequently express more than words, pay close attention to non-verbal cues like body language and facial expressions. By paying close attention while someone is speaking to you, you show that you respect them and that you are eager to understand them on their terms.

Avoid interrupting them when they are speaking to you. Give them your undivided attention, pause what you are doing at the moment, and listen. Try to reduce any distractions. For instance, turn off a blaring television in the background, or if construction is happening outside and there is a ton of noise, close the window. If you are unsure what they are trying to communicate to you, simply repeat what you thought they said back to them or politely ask them to repeat themselves. These are all examples of active listening, and it will help enhance your connection with your loved one tremendously.

POSITIVE FRAMING: THE IMPACT OF POSITIVITY IN COMMUNICATION

This approach emphasizes the importance of employing positive language when caring for your loved one and how simply rephrasing or altering the way we communicate can have a profoundly positive impact on their overall wellbeing. Positive framing may change a situation by adding positivity and fostering opportunities for deep connections

At its core, positive framing simply means focusing on strengths rather than weaknesses. It is a form of communication that is meant to convey an optimistic outlook on life and how to positively navigate the complex nature of communication with a person with dementia. It has already been stated that as dementia progresses, individuals experience an assortment of cognitive, behavioral, and language challenges, and it is essential that we acknowledge these changes without falling into the trap of negativity.

Understanding Positive Framing

This approach involves remaining calm, reassuring, and soothing, and evolving our communication techniques to help encourage and comfort our loved ones. It is important to note that positive language should never be patronizing but should maintain respect and dignity.

Framing statements, requests, or instructions can make your loved ones more receptive and cooperative. Rather than giving stern instructions like "Don't go outside," offer a more encouraging and positive response by saying, "Let's stay inside and enjoy the warmth together today." Simply rephrasing this question provides a greater sense of choice, respecting the person's autonomy and dignity rather than issuing them a command they have no choice but to follow. In addition, instead of being blunt and coming across as controlling or rude, find alternative phrases for your responses. Instead of saying "You're wrong," re-frame the statement to say, "Gran, let's try and understand this together." This response not only reduces the chance for confrontation but also creates a sense of collaboration and belonging.

Positive framing involves presenting information or questions in a way that makes them easier to comprehend. Take the pressure off them; instead of asking, "Do you remember?" which can trigger anxiety if they don't, you can say, "Can you tell me more about that?" This encourages reminiscence without the pressure of recollection.

Furthermore, using familiar and reassuring phrases is invaluable in dementia communication. As the condition progresses, patients often seek solace in the familiar. Employing nicknames they are accustomed to or reminiscing about cherished memories can establish a comforting and positive communication environment. This aids in maintaining their dignity and sense of worth. In addition to aiding in their overall understanding, employing positive framing can help instill empathetic and person-centered care for our loved ones.

Benefits of Positive Framing

There are multiple benefits that individuals with dementia experience when adopting positive framing as a communication technique (Ralph-Savage, 2020):

1. Reduced Anxiety: Both anxiety and agitation are greatly reduced when positive and comforting language is employed.

2. Enhanced Understanding: Using positive phrases and simplified language can reduce confusion and improve comprehension as a result.

3. Enhanced Mood and increased engagement: Positive framing is both encouraging and reassuring, making your loved ones feel comfortable and more willing to engage in conversation or follow instructions.

4. Fostering better relationships: When caregivers adopt positive framing, forming deeper connections with their loved ones becomes far easier.

5. Improved Self-esteem: This form of communication is highly effective in reinforcing your loved one's sense of identity.

6. Enhanced Quality of Life: Contributing to an overall better quality of life by focusing on their strengths and abilities.

7. Smoother Transitions: Positive framing makes difficult adjustments easier and less upsetting as your loved ones feel acknowledged and understood, making conversations more enjoyable and interesting for all involved.

Further Examples and Tips, of Positive Framing

Think carefully about the language you use when speaking to your loved ones. These straightforward positive linguistic modifications can promote a more uplifting and encouraging interactive setting:

- Rather than labeling behavior as "challenging," describe it, such as "frustrated" or "agitated."

- Avoid referring to individuals as "patients" or "victims." Instead, use phrases like "a person living with dementia."

- Replace impersonal and aggressive terms like "handling" with "caring for."

- Replace "You can't drive anymore" with "Why don't we take a walk? It's a beautiful day."

- Instead of saying, "You can't go home," try, "We are home; what do you love most about being here?"

- Avoid telling them they are "wrong" when they make mistakes; encourage them to try again or explore new possibilities.

In essence, we need to be mindful of which words we choose to use, as the right or wrong assortment of words can drastically impact how individuals with dementia respond (Ralph-Savage, 2020).

OVERCOMING COMMUNICATION BARRIERS: STRATEGIES FOR TOUGH DAYS

Unfortunately, given the nature of dementia, there will undoubtedly be some tough days when communication will seem even more challenging than on other days. On these days, communication barriers may seem insurmountable; however, even on these so-called "bad days," there are strategies you can adopt to help make communication less elusive. Two highly effective techniques have been proven to aid in communication during these tough days. These techniques are known as "redirection" and "music memory."

Redirection is employed to distract an individual with dementia if they have become fixated on a specific idea or topic of conversation or display abnormal signs of agitation or nervousness. How redirection works is that we try to direct our loved ones' attention towards a specific activity they love doing, an interest that captivates them, or engaging in a topic of conversation that they love. This will help to diffuse agitation and tension and prevent us from engaging in frustrating and fruitless arguments with no end. Consider this, if your loved one is confused and wants to go "home" to their childhood home, but that is not a feasible option, you could try to distract them by asking them if they would like to paint, as this typically brings them joy and distracts them from the fixation in their minds.

Music memory is another potent tool for communication with your loved one when connecting becomes increasingly difficult. We have already touched on the effects of music being able to stir up memories of the past. These memories are often unaffected, despite the cognitive degenerative effects of dementia. A study conducted by the Alzheimer's Disease Center at Boston University highlights that people with dementia typically retain the ability to retain music memory over time (Boston University, 2021). You can take advantage of this by making a customized playlist with their favorite songs or by using consoling melodies to comfort them when they're upset. When words fail, music, with its capacity to cut through language boundaries, may be perceived as a source of comfort and connection.

CHAPTER 5
THE DAILY ROUTINE: PRACTICAL SKILLS FOR CAREGIVING

We will set out on a journey that will provide us with the tools necessary to offer comfort, maintain independence, and establish a sense of predictability amid dementia as an ever-evolving condition. We will cover all the necessities and basics, ranging from personal care and hygiene to the complexities of medication management, nutrition, and mobility.

We need to understand and adopt practical skills to help navigate the evolving challenges of what being a caregiver truly entails. Acquiring these skills and techniques is not just a necessity to ensure we are providing adequate care to our loved ones but also to provide the often neglected care for ourselves. Additionally, it also serves as a source of remarkable empowerment for those we care for.

THE BASICS OF PERSONAL CARE AND HYGIENE

It is not uncommon for individuals living with dementia to frequently forget to practice personal hygiene or groom themselves regularly. Routine actions like taking a shower and getting dressed often go neglected if not addressed. This can be perplexing and rather upsetting for caregivers and their families. However, there are strategies and techniques caregivers can use to help facilitate personal care for those they are caring for, including routines, gentle reminders, and user-friendly products. Patience is crucial, and respecting their dignity is a must, even in small gestures like providing a robe during bathing.

To further improve their general well-being, keeping their surroundings tidy and welcoming is essential to maintaining familiarity, which will in turn reduce stress and anxiety. Cleaning regularly can prevent further health complications and create an environment that feels tranquil and cozy. Ensuring a safe and comfortable environment with calming colors and recognizable objects lessens disorientation for your loved ones and decreases their resistance toward personal care.

Bathing and Dressing

This is especially humiliating when someone is additionally dealing with incontinence. Thus, it is no surprise that you may be met with resistance when trying to help your loved ones get changed or bathe.

To prevent embarrassment or humiliation, privacy must always be respected. Creating a private space by drawing the blinds and closing the doors, hiding mirrors if they don't recognize themselves, and approaching with patience and assurance are some strategies you can employ to make these processes easier.

Creating a pleasant atmosphere is essential; a bathroom should be cozy, clean, well-lit, and comfortable. Playing soothing music while they are bathing or getting dressed is a fantastic way to create a calming atmosphere in which they can feel relaxed. Furthermore, it's important to respect their former bathing habits, such as what time they usually took their baths and how they liked to enjoy them; for instance, if they used to draw a bubble bath every day at 17:30, then keep it that way. Encouraging self-care and arranging items in sequence helps maintain order and independence.

A technique to make bathing easier for all involved is to simplify the process (Department of Health & Human Services, 2019):

•Offer limited choices, such as asking if they would prefer a bath or a shower, or if they'd like to bathe after dinner or just before bed. This will help them feel like they are in control.

•Let them test the water before entering. You can either pour some water gently over their hands or assist them as they feel the water for themselves.

•Make them feel like they are in charge. Encourage their independence by letting them do as much as they can themselves without assistance; however, be sure to be present in case they need you.

•Categorize items and have a system. Arrange soap, washcloth, towel, and clean clothes in a sequence for easy access during the bathing process.

Additionally, when helping dress your loved one, try to keep the choices to a minimum and provide them with 2 or 3 options of clothes rather than asking them to choose an outfit from their entire wardrobe. This will help them reach a decision much faster, and they will feel in control of making that decision. Caregivers should change their clothes frequently for hygienic purposes, especially if incontinence is something your loved one struggles with. You can also help enhance their self-esteem by subtly praising how they look and admiring their outfit.

Dental Care

Ensuring that your loved one is still having regular dental check-ups is important. However, remember to inform the dentist of your loved ones' condition, as the dentist may face some resistance from them due to the cognitive degeneration and behavioral changes brought upon by dementia.

As the caregiver, you are more than likely going to have to remind your loved one to brush their teeth and floss, especially as the condition progresses into the later stages. Eventually, there is a chance you will have to brush their teeth for them. In this event, sit the person you are caring for on a straight-backed chair while you stand behind them. Support your loved one against your body, gently cradle their head with one arm, and brush their teeth with the other hand using a dry toothbrush and a pea-sized amount of toothpaste. (Alzheimer's Society, 2021)

Shaving, Nail, and Hair Care

Reminders may be required for daily tasks like shaving as dementia progresses. Depending on whether they are used to using electric or conventional razors, supervision may be necessary to reduce the risk of them hurting themselves.

People often forget this, but ear care is something that should not be overlooked. A buildup of earwax could potentially lead to some unnecessary hearing problems if left unattended; however, before doing anything, speak to your loved one's doctor to find out the best course of action to remove the earwax. In addition, you may need to assist your loved ones with maintaining their fingernails or toenails or consider taking them to a beautician.

Lastly, hair care is a sensitive issue and something we often link to our very identity, so it would be advised to schedule routine salon appointments as these can remain highly enjoyable experiences for individuals with dementia.

MANAGING MEDICATIONS: ENSURING PROPER INTAKE

The management of medication can become fairly challenging for those who care for individuals with dementia, particularly as the condition reaches its later stages. The delicate daily routines frequently become confused, resulting in missing important doses or leading to them resisting the medication entirely. There are practical solutions to this problem that can make managing medication intake far smoother.

Pill organizers or daily pill containers, provided by MedCenter and other similar pill-organizing brands, feature weekly or monthly divider sections with distinct markings. Utilizing these pill dividers is an effective strategy, as they make the process of administering pills to your loved one far simpler. You will be able to quickly identify if they have taken their daily dose of medication. You will also be able to prevent them from taking a double dose if they had taken it earlier that day but forgot and now want to take an additional dose (Alzheimer's Association, 2019).

In addition to using pill organizers, you can also make use of technology by setting timely alarms on your digital devices. You can also use devices such as Amazon Echo, Google Nest Mini, Apple HomePod Mini, and the new Sonos Era 100 .

This app will notify you when your loved one needs to take their medication and ensure it is being taken as prescribed by their doctors, reducing the risk of a mishap in dosage or frequency.

If possible, try to involve your loved one in the process of taking their medication, as this will make them feel in control and empower them. Beyond empowerment, it can also limit their reluctance to take the medication in the first place.

As dementia advances into its later stages, more extensive care during the medication process will be required beyond pill organizers, reminders, and a daily routine. In the event of this, try some of these tips:

- Use positive framing, straightforward language, and clear instructions: "Here you go, Mom. This pill helps you with your blood pressure; let's take it together with some water."

- If they refuse to take their medication at that very moment, don't force them; wait an hour or so (if the medication allows it) and try again later.

- If you notice that swallowing is becoming an increasing issue, then ask your doctor if there is an alternative form the medication comes in, such as a liquid syrup.

- To avoid unintentional overdoses, put safety first by keeping your loved one's medication in a secure and locked cabinet or drawer (Alzheimer's Association, 2019).

By implementing these strategies, managing medication will be far smoother and you will be protecting the overall well-being of those you care for in the process.

NUTRITION AND MEALTIME TIPS

While it is essential to ensure your loved ones are sticking to a balanced diet, it becomes increasingly difficult as the disease progresses, as many individuals living with dementia present challenges with the act of eating or exercise a disinterest in food entirely. Our jobs as caregivers are to ensure that their nutritional needs are met, so to simplify mealtimes and make the process run smoothly, consider these tips and tricks throughout the various stages of dementia (Alzheimer's Association, 2022):

Early Stages

1. Establish a Routine: Stick to a schedule and develop regular meal times and intervals to create a consistent routine that your loved ones can get into the habit of executing. Ultimately, this will help reduce confusion around mealtimes.

2. Utilize Contrasting Tableware: Using cutlery and crockery that have high-contrast colors can often help your loved ones distinguish food from their plate, reducing confusion and frustration. There are products available, such as Freedom Dinnerware, that are specifically designed for individuals with cognitive impairment.

3. Patience and encouragement: Always remain calm and patient during mealtimes. Do not rush individuals with dementia while they are eating; instead, offer gentle encouragement if you find they are encountering difficulties during mealtimes.

Middle Stages

1. Introduce Finger Foods into Their Diet: This could be sandwiches, chicken strips, pigs in a blanket, pizza rolls, etc.

THE DAILY ROUTINE: PRACTICAL SKILLS FOR CAREGIVING

By incorporating these finger foods into their diet, you are helping them become more self-serving and independent.

2. Adaptive Tableware: Make use of larger bowls, plates with rims, and utensils with larger handles or even weights to make the process of eating easier and less messy

3. Utilize Non-Skid Surfaces: At mealtimes, place plates and bowls on non-skid surfaces, such as towels or cloths, as this will help reduce spillage

4. Get Cups with Lids and Use Straws: To further reduce spillage and potential burns from hot drinks like tea or coffee, serve liquids in cups with lids and a bendable straw, or if you serve a mug or glass, make sure to only fill it up halfway

Late Stages

1. Allow for Longer Mealtimes: As dementia progresses to its conclusive stages mealtimes can often take more than an hour

2. Make Dining Social: Whenever it is possible encourage social dining as this will not only assist in maintaining connections with others but also act as a motivation to eat.

3. Make food easier to swallow and consume: Grind up or cut food smaller if you find that your loved one is having trouble swallowing. Additionally, make use of soft foods that are high in nutrition such as scrambled eggs, oatmeal, porridge, mashed potatoes, and cottage cheese, as this will make consumption of food easier.

4. Utilize thicker liquids: To minimize the likelihood of chok-ing, offer thicker liquids like shakes, nectars, or thick juices.

5. Monitor Swallowing: Make sure your loved ones sit upright and tilt their heads slightly forward when they eat as this will help prevent choking hazards. You can additionally, politely ask to check their mouth after the meal to confirm that they have swallowed their food, but first get their permission, unless it is an emergency.

6. Prepare their favorite foods: This will help stimulate their appetite and get them excited for mealtime. Consider offering smaller, more frequent meals and if you opt for this approach, make it part of their routine.

7. Be their memory aid: Some individuals may forget if they've eaten. compartmentalize their meal, such as juice, toast, and cereal, to accommodate this.

8. Learn the Heimlich maneuver: It is wise to learn this technique and be vigilant for choking signs at all times, especially in the later stages of dementia.

ESTABLISHING A DAILY ROUTINE: THE POWER OF PREDICTABILITY

Creating a routine for your loved one is possibly the most important aspect of caregiving. This is not the stage in your loved ones' lives where you should be introducing significant changes or "new ways" of doing things. Instead, we should be doing our utmost to develop a routine that is consistent with our loved ones' lifelong habits. For instance, if your loved one habitually has a cup of tea at 1:00 p.m. or enjoys playing cards on a late Sunday morning, uphold these familiar routines.

However, flexibility is paramount, especially as dementia progresses and their cognitive, behavioral, and mobility symptoms start to worsen. We need to be adaptive, calm, and patient. Adapt the routine to accommodate their changing capabilities and newly developed difficulties while still trying your utmost to empower your loved one to do as much as they can on their own to preserve their dignity, self-esteem, independence, and autonomy. The ultimate goal of these routines is to provide structure while fostering an environment void of stress and disorientation. Remember that it is highly likely that you will need to adjust this routine throughout the dementia journey and that is okay. If signs of boredom or irritability begin to present themselves, consider redirecting their attention to another activity, tweaking the routine slightly without losing its structure. Remember, it is also okay to allow for some breaks in between activities.

Another effective technique for instilling routine is inviting your loved ones to help with household chores or activities, this could be asking them if they would like to help wash the dishes or load the dishwasher. Letting them help you fold clothes is another effective technique as this is beneficial for both their cognitive and motor skills. It doesn't matter if the dishes they washed weren't pristinely cleaned or the clothes they folded weren't immaculately folded, let them do their best without correction, and offer some subtle praise once the activity is over to boost their self-esteem. It is crucial to also incorporate mundane yet essential daily activities into their routine such as administering medication, brushing their teeth, bathing, and exercising if their body allows it. Ensure these activities happen around about the same time every day, for example, if they bathe at 4pm try and stick to 4pm being bath time. This helps instill a sense of order and purpose in their day.

Many individuals struggle to comprehend both time and place; thus, we must establish these for them through the utilization of non-verbal cues. If their favorite TV show is at 19:00, turn on the TV to remind them. If they used to love having Sunday roasts with family, make it for them and enjoy the meal with them. Daily rituals such as drawing the curtains in the morning and at night help them distinguish what time of day it is. It may be wise to also make a visual schedule for them on a whiteboard or a marked calendar so they can follow it for themselves or utilize day clocks. Using these non-verbal visual cues to indicate both place and time becomes more prevalent as dementia progresses and verbal communication becomes ever more elusive.

Lastly, add some highlights into their routine for them to look forward to. These could be any activity that is aligned with their interests, such as puzzles, arts and crafts, gardening, knitting, or playing cards. These activities are Both therapeutic and bring delight to their day.

By following these steps, you can create a caregiving routine that fosters a sense of comfort, purpose, and engagement for your loved ones (Where You Live Matters, 2020).

PROMOTING QUALITY SLEEP: TIPS FOR A RESTFUL NIGHT

Many individuals with dementia struggle with sleep disturbances, thus developing a restful sleep routine for your loved ones often poses a significant challenge; however, there are strategies you can adopt to enhance their sleep quality and improve their quality of life in the process.

First and foremost, you need to establish a regular sleep schedule and stick to it, as this will have a pivotal impact on regulating your loved ones' internal body clock. This can be achieved by setting consistent bedtime and wakeup times. This will essentially anchor their circadian rhythms, which will assist in both the process of waking up and falling asleep more naturally.

Another strategy to consider is to create a sleeping environment that is as calm and as void of distractions as possible.

This includes ensuring their room blocks out any excessive light that could disturb their quality of sleep or removing any sounds that could prevent them from falling asleep or disrupting their sleeping patterns. Utilize blackout curtains to shield against any unwanted light and invest in a white noise machine as this will help mask any disruptive background noises that could potentially be disturbing them. It may also be wise to look into getting weighted blankets as these offer a comforting sensation, similar to as if somebody was cuddling or hugging them, which could foster a sense of security and limit unnecessary anxiety.

Be mindful of their caffeine intake. Either reduce the amount of caffeine they consume or eliminate it from their diet entirely, especially any caffeine intake in the late afternoon or evening. Promoting regular physical activity is also effective in helping ensure enhanced sleep quality as it helps your loved ones expend energy and thus become more tired in the evening. However, make sure that all exercises are done in the late morning or early afternoon as strenuous activities too close to bedtime can have the opposite effect.

If sleep disturbances persist after you have tried these strategies, it is best if you seek guidance from their healthcare providers, as it may signal an underlying health concern or a side-effect to one of their medications. If this is the case their neurologist will evaluate the situation and address these issues to ensure your loved ones are receiving the appropriate treatment and support they need to enhance their quality of sleep.

CHAPTER 6
DECODING DEMENTIA BEHAVIORS: A COMPASSIONATE APPROACH

Behavioral changes in individuals with dementia can often be understood as a means of communicating and expressing themselves as their language skills decline. You may witness rather drastic changes in the typical personality or behavior. This is often due to them trying to convey their needs, discomfort, or distress to others.

For instance, someone with dementia might exhibit agitation as a response to pain, hunger, or boredom; however, they struggle to verbally communicate this to anyone. It is important to remember that these behaviors are indications of their discomfort or unfulfilled needs, rather than deliberate behaviors or actions. Understanding this provides caregivers with insight into how to react to these changes in behavior with greater empathy and efficiency. While many of these behaviors are due to frustration when your loved ones are trying to express themselves, it is also important to bear in mind that these alterations in their personality are also due to the degenerative symptoms of dementia as a whole.

Some of the common behavior changes that you can expect to see in your loved ones include aggression, wandering, restlessness, paranoia, and sundowning. Let's look at what these behavior changes imply and how we can help (Logan, 2016).

AGGRESSION AND AGITATION

Agitation is a term used to describe a variety of dementia-related behaviors, such as irritation, sleep disturbances, and aggression (both verbal and non-verbal). Your loved one's agitation and aggression can be triggered due to a variety of variables, including fear, an inability to express themselves, physical discomfort or sleeplessness, and unfamiliar environmental factors. The most common cause of agitation and aggression in people living with dementia is when they feel that control and autonomy are being taken away from them.

Consider these strategies to both prevent aggression and agitation as well as soothe these behaviors if they arise:

• Reduce the number of people in one room and eliminate noise or clutter

• Maintain familiarity and stick to a routine. Don't rearrange furniture or move household objects out of their designated spaces. Familiarity such as cherished items and photographs helps provide a sense of security and can even spark pleasant memories from the past.

•Reduce caffeine and sugar, as these spike energy levels and can make them feel overwhelmed

• Keep any dangerous objects locked away or out of reach

• You may engage in gentle touch, play soothing music, or suggest going for a walk with them to try and mitigate their agitation. Always speak in a soft and reassuring voice, and never resort to restraining them, as you can severely injure them.

- Let them feel in control. Encourage them to do as much as they can by themselves, as this will preserve their indepen-dence and allow them to feel in charge.

- Acknowledge their confusion or anger; do not tell them they are being inappropriate; they are not doing this by choice.

- Redirecting your loved one's attention to a calming activity or changing their environment can help diffuse aggressive behaviors. For example, ask if they want to play Scrabble or if they want to paint

SUNDOWNING

It is common for confusion, agitation, disorientation, restless-ness, and other challenging behaviors to intensify in the later hours of the day, particularly late afternoon and at night. This phenomenon is known as "sundowning" and is under-stood to be caused by several combined factors, such as hunger, pain, not enough exposure to sunlight, overstimula-tion during the day, tiredness, and disruptions of their internal body clock, which often lead to your loved ones getting confused between day and night (Alzheimer's Soci-ety, 2021).

Consider these strategies to help manage sundowning behavior:

- Encourage more daytime activities, especially physical activity, and discourage naps or other forms of inactivity.

- Monitor diet. Limit excess sugar, caffeine, and unhealthy snacks such as "junk food" earlier in the day. Make sure your loved ones have smaller, lighter meals before they go to bed.

- During the afternoon and evening, provide a relaxed and structured environment with activities like leisurely walks outside, card games, or calming music to soothe them and keep them occupied.

- Utilize ample lighting before sunset and ensure the curtains are drawn at dusk, as this will reduce the amount of shadow, which will help ease confusion. Make use of nightlights in your loved ones' bedroom as well as in the hallway, kitchen, and bathroom.

- To ensure safety and reduce the risk of your loved ones injuring themselves, block stairs with gates, secure the kitchen, and make sure all dangerous items are out of reach

- Remember, you need to take care of yourself too. We can't care for others if we are failing to care for ourselves. Prioritize your sleep as a caregiver. It may be wise to ask for assistance now and again from your friends, family, or even a hired professional to ensure you are getting quality rest yourself, including power naps during the day if required.

WANDERING

Many individuals engage in aimless wandering as a result of restlessness and confusion, which is particularly common in the middle and latter stages of dementia.your loved ones may be driven to wander around due to various factors. Wandering often stems from your loved one's basic needs; they could be hungry or thirsty, or they could be looking for the bathroom, but getting confused and lost along the way. Additionally, they may wander off somewhere because they are fixated on finding somebody, often somebody who has long since passed, like their mother or father, for instance. Other common red flags for potential wandering can include repeated pacing or becoming anxious in social gatherings or a crowd. Identifying the root causes for wandering becomes challenging as it can be one of many variables; however, if you can spot these signs in advance, they hold valuable insights for managing this behavior in your loved one.

Consider these strategies to reduce the risk of wandering (Alzheimer's Association, 2019b):

- Encourage structured and meaningful activities throughout the day to keep them busy and occupied. This could include activities like helping with laundry or preparing a meal with you
- Identify what time of day the risk of wandering is most likely, particularly if they suffer from sundowning, and plan activities during those hours that effectively keep them entertained and engaged
- Make sure that your loved one's basic needs are always being met, such as meals, hydration, and going to the bathroom
- Offer reassurance to your loved one if you notice they are feeling confused or disoriented
- Keep car keys or house keys out of reach, especially if it is no longer safe for them to drive
- Avoid overwhelming crowds that could cause disorientation and anxiety, such as bustling malls
- Monitor how your loved ones respond to new surroundings and do not leave them unsupervised in unfamiliar environments (Alzheimer's Association , 2019b).

As dementia progresses, so does the urge to wander; thus, it is wise to prepare your home or wherever your loved one is staying to reduce the risk of wandering as their condition worsens. Consider these tips and tricks:

- Place deadbolts out of the line of sight on exterior doors (high or low) without locking your loved one in.
- Install night lights throughout your home
- Use childproof locks
- Install safety gates
- Remove tripping hazards.
- Hide doors with removable curtains or screens.
- Utilize warning bells above your doors and install monitoring devices that will alert you when a door has been opened
- Use pressure-sensitive mats by the door or bedside for movement alerts
- Label room doors to alleviate confusion
- Never leave your loved one alone in a car, even if you are at home

Lastly, it's important to plan. The tremendous stress that caregivers and family members experience when their loved one wanders off is extremely emotionally taxing and a hazard to your health. Thus, it is wise to have a plan in place before your loved one potentially wanders off somewhere. Here's what you can do:

- You can enroll your loved one in a wandering response service, which is specifically in place for situations like these
- Politely ask your neighbors, friends, and other family members to be on the lookout for your loved one wandering, or request that they report back to you immediately if they have spotted your loved one wandering.

- Always keep a recent and close-up photo of your loved one on your phone, in your wallet, or in your phone case for identification purposes

- Make a list of all the potential places they could have wandered off to, such as former residences or workplaces, their favorite restaurant, the church or their designated place of worship, or the hairdresser, etc.

Wandering is an incredibly stressful ordeal for everyone involved; thus, it is critical that we remain vigilant and put these strategies in place before a situation escalates .

SEEKING PROFESSIONAL HELP

Caring for an individual with dementia can at times be a formidable and overwhelming task, despite our best efforts to provide quality care. As caregivers, it is crucial for us to acknowledge the importance of seeking external assistance when necessary, whether from medical professionals, support groups, counseling services, or our network of family and friends.

It is extremely valuable to establish a pattern of routine checkups with your loved ones neurologists and other doctors who are caring for them These specialists are qualified to thoroughly evaluate your loved ones' behavior, provide helpful advice, and modify treatment plans as and if required.

Additionally, it is important to consider support groups and counseling services for your emotional well-being. These groups establish a sense of community and understanding where caregivers can share similar experiences and difficulties in a safe environment. These will not only help provide you with emotional support but will also equip you with practical advice to help you navigate the complexities of dementia caregiving. Always remember that seeking help or asking for assistance is not a sign of weakness but rather a proactive step towards providing your loved one and yourself with the care and support you both deserve, and at times it is often the responsible action to take.

SHARE YOUR HEART, SHARE YOUR REVIEW

"*When we give cheerfully and accept gratefully, everyone is blessed.*" - **Maya Angelou**

Did you know that the most beautiful gifts in life are those that we give without expecting anything in return? That's something I've learned on this journey of caregiving, and I'm excited to share it with you.

I have a small but meaningful request for you...

Would you be willing to help a fellow traveler on the path of caregiving, even if you never meet them?

Imagine someone just like you, embarking on this challenging yet rewarding journey of Dementia Caregiving. They might feel lost, overwhelmed, and in need of guidance – feelings that you might have experienced too.

My goal is to make the journey of Dementia Caregiving an open book for everyone. Every step I take is towards fulfilling this goal. And to achieve it, I need to reach out to... well, everyone.

That's where your role becomes vital. People often rely on the experiences of others when choosing a book (yes, they do judge a book by its cover and its reviews!). So, here's my heartfelt request on behalf of a caregiver you haven't met yet:

Please consider leaving a review for this book.

It doesn't cost anything, and it takes less than a minute, but your words have the power to change another caregiver's life. Your review could be the beacon of hope that...

...guides one more caregiver in their journey. ...supports a family navigating through dementia care. ...offers invaluable advice to someone in need. ...inspires another heart to find strength and resilience. ...turns another challenging story into a story of triumph.

To experience the joy of helping and to make a real difference, all you need to do is take a brief moment to leave a review.

Please use the QR code on the next page to share your thoughts:

If the idea of supporting a fellow caregiver warms your heart, then you are exactly the kind of person who belongs in our community. Welcome to the club. You are now one of us.

I am thrilled to continue guiding you on your caregiving journey. The insights and experiences that await you in the next chapters are something I am eager for you to discover.

Thank you from the deepest part of my heart. Now, let's get back to our journey together.

With gratitude,

Mary Ann Martin

SHARE YOUR HEART, SHARE YOUR REVIEW

CHAPTER 7
NAVIGATING THE EMOTIONAL LABYRINTH: STRATEGIES FOR DEALING WITH STRESS, GUILT, AND BURNOUT

Caregiving for our loved ones is a rewarding journey; however, it also comes with a set of emotional challenges. We will delve into the emotional landscape of the role of a caregiver and equip you with the insight and invaluable strategies you will need to navigate that landscape. These strategies will help you deal with overwhelming stress, lingering guilt, and the ever-present risk of caregiver burnout.

We will learn how to prioritize your own emotional and physical health needs, in addition to providing the best care for your loved ones. We will highlight the importance of self-care.

UNDERSTANDING THE EMOTIONAL ROLLERCOASTER: THE IMPACT OF CAREGIVING ON YOUR EMOTIONS

As caregivers, we often go through a rollercoaster of emotions when we are caring for our loved ones; these range from overwhelming stress, frustration, ambivalence, anger, anxiety, indifference, irritability, fear, grief, guilt, loneliness, loss, tiredness, frustration, and even resentment from time to time. These feelings are all completely normal and come with the territory of being a caregiver. They are not something you should be ashamed of ; instead, it is best if you recognize and validate these feelings rather than ignore or suppress them.

These feelings can all be attributed to a phenomenon known as caregiver burnout. Caregiver burnout is a state of profound physical, emotional, and mental exhaustion that often shifts our typical compassionate attitudes to those of a negative one. Burnout is often attributed to a lack of support or trying to carry out too many responsibilities for one person to handle effectively. These responsibilities are physical, emotional, and financial (WebMD, 2011).

In addition, many caregivers suffer from illogical or unwarranted guilt when they prioritize their own needs ahead of those of their loved ones. Feelings of confinement and the difficulty of coping with behavioral changes in their loved ones make this emotional stress and exhaustion worse. Remember, it is okay to put yourself first now and again, as your well-being is a priority as well. It is also okay to feel overwhelmed, as caregiving is an extremely taxing job that often tests our limits beyond what we can take. Be kind to yourself and work through these emotions; don't suppress them and allow them to manifest into issues that are even more severe. Be kind to yourself.

Neglecting caregiver burnout can lead to a cascade of symptoms that significantly impact your overall well-being and can similarly present themselves as clinical depression; below are some signs to look out for (WebMD, 2011).
- sudden lack of interest in hobbies and activities that you once loved

- persisting feelings of overwhelming sadness, helplessness, hopelessness, and irritability
- poor sleep quality owing to disrupted sleep patterns
- compromised immunity
- consistent feelings of being emotionally and physically drained
- a significantly elevated risk of using alcohol, narcotics, or sleep medication as a crutch
- severely negative thoughts as well as suicidal thoughts
- the occasional thought of harming the individual you are caring for

If caregiver burnout is ignored, it can result in severe consequences for your well-being; thus, it is of the utmost importance that you not only acknowledge your emotions but also take proactive steps to address them.

STRATEGIES FOR MANAGING STRESS: HOW TO STAY CALM IN THE CHAOS

The emotional and physical demands of caregiving can overwhelm and deter even the strongest individuals out there. Luckily, there are many strategies one can adopt to help reduce the risk of caregiver burnout and the overwhelming challenges that come with it. Remember that taking care of yourself is just as important as taking care of those you love; if you fail to look after your well-being, you won't be able to provide care to anybody else.

Consider these tips to prioritize your well-being and counteract the effects of caregiver stress (Alzheimer's Society, 2019):

NAVIGATING THE EMOTIONAL LABYRINTH: STRATEGIES FOR DEALING WITH STRESS, GUILT, AND BURNOUT

1. Learn as much as you can about dementia stress: By acquiring the necessary knowledge about dementia and the comprehensive care strategies that come with it, you will gain invaluable insight that will help prepare yourself as you navigate the complexities of the dementia journey. Being armed with this knowledge will provide you with a comprehensive understanding of the challenges you can expect to face and foster your ability to adapt as dementia progresses through the stages.

2. Utilize Relaxation Techniques: Four highly effective relaxation techniques will help ease caregiver burnout if done regularly. The first of these techniques is visualization. This is achieved by mentally picturing a place or situation that is calm and peaceful; this could be a tranquil beach, a lush forest, or perhaps mentally revisiting a memory that you cherish. The second of these techniques is meditation. Try and incorporate this into your routine every day for about 15 minutes to let go of stressful thoughts weighing you down. Next is to practice breathing exercises; simply slow your breathing when you feel stressed and focus on taking slower and deeper breaths till you calm down. Lastly, make use of progressive muscle relaxation, which is when you tighten and then relax each of your muscle groups. Start at one end of your body and slowly work your way to the other end (Alzheimer's Association, 2023).

3. Make exercise part of your daily routine: This doesn't have to take a large chunk of your day; it can even be as short as ten to fifteen minutes a day. These exercises can be any form of physical activity as long as you are moving and staying active, as this will help reduce stress and improve your overall well-being. Try and make these exercises something you enjoy doing, as this will motivate you to be consistent. This could be anything: gardening, yoga, dancing, or palates.

4. Be realistic about the progressive nature of dementia: The reality is that dementia is a progressive disease and will become gradually more severe regardless of the quality of our care. This may be disheartening, but acknowledging these challenges and changes helps us better adjust our expectations as time passes

5. Be realistic about yourself: You need to recognize that you are not Superman or Superwoman. No matter how much we want to be them, we aren't. You can only do so much. Do not beat yourself up over the bad days, and do not blame yourself if the dementia symptoms of your loved ones become more severe; it is not your fault. You are doing your best, so try and focus on all the value you have brought to the lives of your loved ones instead of everything else that is out of your control.

6. Set boundaries now and again: This might mean saying no to additional responsibilities or scheduling regular breaks from caregiving.

7. Prioritize self-care: This can include getting enough sleep, eating a healthy diet, making time to see the doctor, pampering yourself with a manicure or a message, making time for a social life, and finding time to do activities you love.

8. Seeking support from others: Whether it's family, friends, or a support group, it can help you feel less isolated and provide a safe space to share your experiences and feelings. The more your family and friends are informed about what you are feeling and how you are coping, the better they will be able to support you.

9. Remember to laugh: While dementia is a serious condition, it does not mean we can't look for the brighter side of situations and find solace in laughter. Humor is a fantastic coping mechanism and one we should never abandon.

10. Plan for the Future: Preparing plans may help alleviate some of the stress you may be feeling. If at all possible, go over finances with your loved ones and make plans together accordingly. Future health and personal care decisions should be carefully researched and documented. In addition, it may be wise to talk about legal and estate planning and, if at all possible, involve your loved ones in this discussion.

COPING WITH GUILT: UNDERSTANDING AND OVERCOMING CAREGIVER GUILT

Caregivers often carry the heavy weight of unwarranted and often illogical guilt on their shoulders when they feel that no matter how noble their efforts are, their loved ones are still struggling with dementia. This is by no means the fault of the caregiver or their ability, but a misconception. Often, the stress becomes so overwhelming that we respond by holding ourselves accountable for our loved ones struggling and their symptoms becoming progressively worse. This sense of guilt can amplify the inherent stress of the caregiving role and can become an incredibly taxing and mentally unhealthy ordeal if left unattended. Caregivers can experience guilt even when they are performing exceptionally well. The truth is, we can't cure dementia, and we often wish we could.

One of the primary reasons for guilt is resentment over lost time. We feel guilty at times, as we sometimes blame our loved ones for all the time we have lost in our own lives. When you spend so much of your time caring for others, it's common to feel as though you're missing out on other aspects of your life, such as your dreams, hobbies, social life, career advancements, and love life. Often, caregivers believe they should not be feeling this way; however, it is completely normal to hold some resentment, but remember that you are not resentful of your loved one; you are resentful of dementia itself.

Unresolved issues from the past, such as prior arguments before your loved ones got diagnosed with dementia or childhood trauma, can often leave caregivers feeling weighed down with guilt as they believe these issues will never be resolved. The truth is, they can be resolved, but do not wait to resolve them. Resolve any issues you have with your loved ones in the early stages of dementia before it is too late because the weight of these issues can make the caregiving journey even more emotionally demanding.

Resist the urge to compare yourself with other caregivers. It is human nature to compare ourselves, but it rarely ends in a positive outcome. Comparing ourselves to other caregivers will likely trigger guilt within us, as we may perceive ourselves as inadequate because we believe we may never measure up to the "remarkable" abilities of other caregivers.

Another factor of guilt that falls heavily on the shoulders of caregivers is the realization that they may have to place their loved ones in assisted living or nursing homes. This stirs up guilt within us as we grapple with feelings of failure or abandonment when we are forced to make these difficult decisions. However, the truth is that as dementia progresses to its conclusive stages, symptoms can become so severe that we cannot provide our loved ones with the care they deserve that other facilities can.

Finally, personal health problems, both mental and physical, can compound this feeling of guilt. For instance, if you are suffering from anxiety and depression as a result of watching your loved ones progressively get worse before your eyes,

NAVIGATING THE EMOTIONAL LABYRINTH: STRATEGIES FOR DEALING WITH STRESS, GUILT, AND BURNOUT

you may feel like you are being selfish to seek help or have bad days, as it will take up time that you could be using to care for your loved one. This is incredibly unhealthy and will only do a disservice to yourself and those you care for.

While caregiver grief, burnout, and stress are extremely common, there are several techniques and strategies you can adopt to reduce the risk of feeling this way (Brown, 2023):

1. Acknowledge the guilt: Don't ignore what you are feeling; rather, identify it and accept that feeling guilty is part of the territory of being a caregiver from time to time. Recognizing and acknowledging your emotions is the first step to effectively managing them.

2. Never forget the bigger picture: Though certain situations can feel arduous and extremely stressful, keep in mind that they are temporary and will not last forever. Reflect on the sacrifices you make for your loved one and recognize the value of your caregiving efforts.

3. We're humans; we make mistakes. Understand that no one is perfect, and it's okay to make mistakes. Try to forgive yourself and focus on all the good things you're doing for your loved one. This is not something you can simply ignore and you need to constantly remind yourself that you are doing the best that you can

4. Prioritize some time for yourself. yourself You matter too: This is something we often forget as caregivers. It is crucial to dedicate some time to yourself; otherwise, you will burn out and even risk compromising your overall well-being.

5. Trust yourself. You've got this: Don't doubt yourself, and believe whatever actions you take are in the best interest of those you care for. Remember, dementia is forever evolving, so our decisions will need to adapt accordingly. Thus, sometimes we will need to make proactive decisions to ensure the future well-being of those we love. They may not agree at first, but trust yourself and understand that these types of decisions are made with their best interests at heart.

6. **Don't hesitate to seek support.** Reach out to family, friends, caregiver support groups, or a psychologist. This does not mean that you are weak or that you have failed; quite the contrary, it often takes a braver person to seek help than those who don't. Whatever support systems you choose to reach out to, they will help you navigate and work through your emotions, particularly your feelings of guilt. You are not alone on this caregiving journey. There are support structures out there that are readily available; you just need to seek them out.

SEEKING PROFESSIONAL HELP: WHEN TO CONSULT A MENTAL HEALTH PROFESSIONAL

As we have mentioned before, caring for a loved one with dementia can bring a plethora of challenges and stress to caregivers and family members. In most cases, caregivers are typically family members without any formal training in caregiving, as it might be difficult to afford professional caregivers on an ongoing basis and there are limited facilities that offer care for dementia patients.

Due to a lack of training or formal experience, these family members take on an enormous task that they are often ill-prepared for. As dementia progresses through its stages of severity, leading to more aggressive degrees of cognitive degeneration and behavioral changes, this daunting task becomes even more challenging to manage. This often leads to overwhelming stress, and studies have found that family caregivers are at far greater risk of experiencing health complications, depression, and anxiety as a result. If feelings of stress, guilt, or burnout become overwhelming, it may be wise to seek professional help. A mental health professional can provide strategies for managing these feelings and provide much-needed support.

Specialized therapists and counselors who focus on caregiver stress and grief offer invaluable guidance and coping strategies tailored to the emotional challenges of caregiving. They will provide you with the insights and tools you need to manage the emotional journey of caregiving effectively, which often proves extremely beneficial in assisting with the unique and stressful challenges they face daily. So whether you are feeling overwhelmed with feelings of grief, stress, or even resentment, seeking psychological support can make a tremendous difference in improving your ability to provide empathetic and quality care for those you care for while still prioritizing your emotional well-being in the process.

Similarly, there is another form of therapy that has been proven to be effective in easing the emotional challenges caregivers commonly face. This is known as cognitive-behavioral therapy (CBT). CBT is a form of therapy that helps family caregivers, with no prior experience, find the coping mechanisms they need to manage difficult circumstances and improve their thinking patterns and behaviors. CBT is highly effective in assisting family caregivers to manage negative and dysfunctional thoughts and find greater enjoyment in their day-to-day activities. For instance, by refocusing their thoughts and realizing that it's neither their fault nor their loved one's fault, caregivers can combat their frustration when dealing with challenging behaviors. By shifting their perspective, caregivers may find it easier to accept their current situation and recognize how much value they bring to their loved ones' lives.

CBT therapy has shown extremely positive results when it comes to addressing mood disorders in caregivers such as depression, anxiety, frustration, and caregiver burnout. You can schedule a CBT session via various formats, including group, online, telephonic, and in-person therapy. The primary aim of this form of therapy is to essentially help caregivers acknowledge, work through, and alleviate emotional, physical, and psychological symptoms so that they can not only improve their quality of life but also enhance their ability to care for those they love (Kwon et al., 2017).

Remember, you should never hesitate to seek help if you're feeling overwhelmed or burned out. It's not a sign of weakness but rather an important step in prioritizing your well-being.

CHAPTER 8
FINDING STRENGTH IN NUMBERS: BUILDING YOUR SUPPORT NETWORK

A ray of hope and resiliency emerges in the form of essential support networks that caregivers can access. New obstacles to caregiving can begin to emerge as dementia steadily progresses to its more severe stages. We will emphasize the fundamental necessity of creating a strong support system and the crucial role it plays in the caregiving journey for everyone involved as we move through this trying phase of our lives.

The value and knowledge support groups offer, along with the emotional comfort they provide, make them the perfect haven for caregivers experiencing burnout. We will discover the power of compassionate connections, unwavering understanding, and fortitude to weather the storms of this progressively aggressive condition.

THE VALUE OF A SUPPORT NETWORK

Caregiving can often feel like an isolating journey, which is why it is paramount to understand that you are not dealing with these challenges on your own. In the USA alone, there are over 34 million family caregivers who are providing unpaid care for their loved ones who are over the age of 50, while nearly 16 million of these caregivers are assisting individuals who have been diagnosed with some variant of dementia (Family Caregiver Alliance, 2016).

These statistics indicate just how essential a role caregiving support groups play in the realm of caregiving as they create a community of individuals in similar situations, thus issuing a lifeline of shared understanding and empathy for the countless individuals going through the caregiving journey.

These support groups offer caregivers a haven where they can freely express their emotions, challenges, and experiences without fear of judgment, thus fostering a profound sense of connection and therapeutic healing. In addition to creating a non-judgmental space, these support groups are essential pillars to offer caregivers the strength, encouragement, and advice they need to remain emotionally resilient during the toughest moments of their caregiving journey.

This understanding and solidarity within the caregiver community are invaluable lifelines that alleviate feelings of isolation and provide solace in times of need. Engaging with those who truly understand the complexities of your journey may considerably reduce stress, validate your experiences, minimize feelings of loneliness, provide you with a sense of connection, and offer unshakable support when you need it most.

Studies have found the significant benefits of caregiving support networks

A study funded by the National Institute on Aging (NIA) and the National Institute of Nursing Research (NINR) involved a sample group of 642 caregivers. These caregivers were offered assistance in the form of interventions such as home visits and telephonic support. The results from this study highlighted that these interventions enhanced these caregiver's quality of life, in addition to reducing their risk of suffering from depressive symptoms. This study also found that there was a significantly lower rate of institutionalization for care recipients as a result of these interventions.

Furthermore, New York University conducted a similar study and found that caregiver support programs were highly effective in delaying the need for nursing home placements for care recipients, delaying placements into these facilities by approximately 1.5 years.

These studies emphasize the immense value that caregiving interventions play in enhancing the well-being of both caregivers and their loved ones (National Institute of Health, 2015).

Support Networks offer a plethora of benefits

Support networks for caregivers are invaluable lifelines, offering relief, guidance, and emotional support. They alleviate the emotional and physical toll of caregiving, enhance our overall well-being, and foster a sense of community and understanding. There are many benefits to support networks, such as: (Daily Caring, 2023).

1.Mitigates the feelings of isolation, loneliness, and fear of judgment: They offer a sense of community and understanding. They provide a secure, accepting environment where caregivers can openly communicate their perspectives, anxieties, and sentiments. Ultimately, helping caregivers feel less overwhelmed and isolated.

2.Reduces the risk of depression, anxiety, and overall mental shutdown: These networks offer caregivers solace in an extremely challenging period of their lives through therapy, emotional support, and resources to aid them in navigating their emotional challenges. They are crucial in maintaining their overall mental well-being by mitigating and reducing symptoms of depression, anxiety, and distress.

3.**Empowers Caregivers:** These groups empower caregivers by arming them with valuable insight and practical solutions. With the knowledge and tools they gain from these groups, they can execute their responsibilities with a greater sense of confidence and improve their sense of control in challenging situations.

4.**Acquire an assortment of valuable coping techniques to enhance their future expectations:** Due to the stressful nature of caregiving, it is no surprise if you experience a rollercoaster of emotions. These support structures teach you the vital coping strategies you need to manage these damaging emotions and adapt to challenges more effectively. In addition, they also prepare you with what to expect in the future by assisting caregivers with a plan for what is to come throughout their caregiving journey.

5.**Become a better caregiver:** As mentioned, one of the primary benefits of these support groups is connecting you with other caregivers. You can learn about tried-and-tested practical advice and tips from your peers that can ease your daily caregiving tasks. They can also share information about helpful resources, such as dementia-friendly activities in your local area or financial aid options.

6.**Serves as a source of respite Care:** Having a robust support network also often means they can help take a load of responsibilities off your back once in a while through respite care. They can step in to provide temporary care, giving you time to rest and recharge. In addition, it also offers assistance in the event of an emergency, providing an extra layer of security and peace of mind.

TYPES OF SUPPORT GROUPS: CHOOSING WHAT SUITS YOU BEST

In the world of caregiving, support groups play a profound role in safeguarding our mental health and aid in navigating the complexities of dementia, however, there are a few varying types of support groups out there. So the question we often ask ourselves is "Which one is right for us?"

When considering the different types of support groups three immediately come to mind, these are in-person, online, and disease-specific support groups.

IN-PERSON SUPPORT GROUPS

These types of support groups provide us with the valuable opportunity to benefit from human interaction by fostering tangible connections in a community made up of fellow caregivers in our local areas. This is extremely valuable, as it provides us with a platform to thrive in an environment of mutual understanding and support. These face-to-face interactions act as a haven where we can freely express anything we would like to share with the group without any judgment, such as our emotions, challenges, concerns, and even our triumphs which can lead to forming lasting friendships with other participants as a result.

However, what is often even more beneficial is when these in-person support groups invite guest speakers such as medical professionals, legal experts, and other thought leaders in the realm of caregiving who can offer incredibly beneficial advice, insight, and perspective. Inviting guest speakers to these kinds of support groups is common practice, and provides an educational aspect over and above the emotional support the group naturally provides. These guest speakers greatly enhance caregiver's knowledge and equip them with the essential tools they need to navigate their roles more effectively (Mayo Clinic, 2021).

Another major benefit of these groups is that they understand how essential it is to balance both your responsibilities as a caregiver and your personal life. Thus, in-person support groups will routinely plan social activities and provide respite care for your loved ones, so caregivers have a chance to destress, socialize, and find joy in shared experiences.

In essence, in-person support groups are a holistic approach to caregiving support. It addresses emotional, educational, and social needs by fostering a warm and empathetic community of similar backgrounds.

DISEASE-SPECIFIC SUPPORT GROUPS

This valuable type of support group offers participants the opportunity to garner specialized knowledge and understanding of particular variants of dementia. Disease-specific support groups are more inclined to provide informational and educational support to caregivers, rather than emphasizing a social or community-based level of support.

Essentially, this support group will furnish tailored information and advice that is aligned specifically to your loved ones' specific challenges with dementia, thus ensuring you have the tools you need to care for your loved one's unique challenges.

These groups are exceptionally beneficial, especially for rarer forms of dementia where information is more scarce. This is because they provide caregivers with access to educational resources and connect them directly with professionals who will arm them with additional insight to provide optimal care and support for their loved ones.

ONLINE SUPPORT GROUPS

Another alternative to consider is online support groups; however, they are not as ideal as in-person support groups or disease-specific support groups. However, they can still be highly valuable if it is not possible to attend the other aforementioned support groups due to distance, transportation, or scheduling constraints or conflicts. They are particularly beneficial in situations where caregivers are facing unique challenges, such as rare conditions or rare variants of dementia, where other caregivers are scattered around the globe. The primary benefit of this type of support group is that it provides you with 24/7 access to forums and chat rooms where you can share your experiences or ask for advice. In addition to hosting regular webinars or virtual events, it also enables you to gain knowledge from the comfort of your home.

However, keep in mind that utilizing online support groups comes with several challenges. Often, participants may find it difficult to interpret body language or facial expressions, and it is often far more challenging to foster a sense of community online. As a result, this often diminishes the richness and depth of communication, which are essential elements to the structure of any support group. The absence of physical presence and tangible human connection can potentially lead to less engagement among participants. Due to the nature of an online environment, the extent to which participants can convey warmth and empathy to others in the group becomes limited, which is another vital component of an effective support group.

Lastly, we cannot ignore that there could potentially be a risk of technical issues, a lack of connectivity, or distractions that could greatly disrupt the sharing of sensitive stories. Therefore, while online support groups are beneficial for caregivers who have busy schedules or live in remote areas, it is more beneficial to participate in in-person and disease-specific support groups if you have the opportunity to do so (Hoy, 2021).

UTILIZING PROFESSIONAL CARE SERVICES

Beyond support groups and therapeutic options, caregivers can also access a medley of dementia-specific care services to help lift the weight of the responsibilities that we have taken on. These services come in the form of in-home, day-to-day, respite, residential, and long-term care services. Additionally, adult daycare centers and end-of-life support such as hospice care are also available.

Collectively, these services act as a comprehensive support network, each providing unique benefits at different stages of dementia. These services have proven to be essential in providing caregivers with the support they need as well as providing their loved ones with the quality care they require.

In-home Care Services

These services offer caregivers invaluable assistance in executing everyday activities, which has proven to be essential in reducing the risk of caregivers experiencing burnout. These services send trained professionals to your home to execute activities such as dressing, bathing, toileting, medication management, and eating, thus lightening the load for caregivers by providing essential support.

Furthermore, these professionals will also assist in filling up your loved one's days with dementia-friendly activities to keep them engaged, entertained, and occupied. These activities often include arts and crafts, gardening, light exercise, puzzles, games, and short walks to name a few. Their assistance will enhance your loved one's well-being and ensure a safe and comfortable home environment for them while giving them the necessary time to rest and recuperate. However, it is important to note that hiring an in-home caregiver every day can be incredibly costly, and often family members take on this role completely unpaid. Although, what you can do is hire these professionals once a week or twice a month, or whatever your budget allows just to give you a chance to come up for air and offer you some respite care (Alzheimers.gov, 2022).

Adult day Centers

Adult day centers are similar to in-home care services as they both offer essential day-to-day support and respite care. However, unlike in-home care services, adult day centers provide a far more social environment for your loved one and get them out of the house for a bit for a change of scenery. Adult day centers are a lifeline for caregivers, as these wonderful services offer your loved ones short-term care in a safe environment where they can socialize and engage in a structured routine filled with activities tailored to improve their cognitive abilities. Not only is this fantastic for their overall well-being, but it also gives them time to take care of themselves and focus on their personal life for the day.

Long-Term Residential Care

This type of care service is generally reserved for individuals who are living with more advanced stages of dementia. Residential care homes offer round-the-clock care and are designed to be long-term care solutions. However, caregivers can have peace of mind knowing that their loved ones are receiving quality care, as these homes are equipped with specially trained staff attuned to the unique needs of each individual staying there.

As dementia progresses, the need for this type of care service becomes increasingly essential as your loved ones will require constant supervision, something you often cannot provide, no matter how much you want to.

Other options you may want to consider include assisted living facilities which are most suitable for the early stages of dementia, while nursing homes offer quality care for individuals who can no longer safely live at home, even with a family caregiver. Another alternative is to consider retirement communities that offer flexible, multi-level care options. Essentially, this means that as their condition worsens, they can gradually move up through the levels of care that they require.

Hospice Care

This is a form of end-of-life care that is designed to make our loved ones as comfortable as possible in their final months or weeks. Hospice care is typically focused on managing pain, symptoms, and side-effects and to allow our loved ones to pass with peace and dignity (Alzheimers.gov, 2022).

REACHING OUT: HOW TO ASK FOR AND ACCEPT HELP

Caregiving is a 24/7 job and can often become a grueling and arduous responsibility to take on even among those with exceptional dedication and deep compassion. However, we don't have to bear the weight of caregiving on our own; there is nothing wrong with seeking out some assistance from friends, family members, and neighbors from time to time to share the load and reduce the risk of succumbing to caregiver burnout.

Requesting help now and then does not translate to you giving up on your loved one or signify any lack of love. Rather, it is a preventative measure to alleviate mental shutdowns. Asking for help is essential for your overall well-being, so you can return to your duties as a well-rested, determined, and more rejuvenated caregiver when you pick up these responsibilities again (Watson, 2022).

However, we often make our lives harder for ourselves by refusing to ask others for assistance with our loved ones. Here are a few reasons why:

- We don't want to be viewed as a bother in the eyes of others.

- We often feel guilty if we cannot personally fulfill all of the needs of our loved ones.

- We're afraid of being told "no."

- We often don't know what kind of assistance is reasonable to request.

Remember, these are not strangers that you will be requesting assistance from; these are people you most likely trust and love, including your friends, family, and even your neighbors.

It is likely they have some degree of understanding regarding your situation and will be more than happy to help out every once in a while. You won't get any help if you don't ask.

In the early stages of dementia, you will probably require far less assistance, as your loved ones will most likely still be able to cope with everyday activities such as driving, entertaining themselves, eating, regular self-care tasks, and some may even still be working. Keep in mind that as dementia progresses, more extensive care is required, and they will likely need help with basic tasks such as eating, walking, self-care, toileting, keeping them occupied, and other day-to-day tasks. It is at this point that you will start to experience the taxing emotional toll of caregiving and become more susceptible to burnout. Thus, you will need to request help from those you love and trust every once in a while when these advanced stages of dementia present themselves.

If you're wondering when it is appropriate to ask for assistance consider these signs and if you are experiencing any of them or a mixture of them then it is probably the right time to be requesting help from those you love before your well-being gets compromised (Watson, 2022).

- Your social life is becoming ever-elusive. Time spent with family and friends is becoming scarcer and scarcer.

- You are losing interest in activities and hobbies that you once loved and are presenting some depressive symptoms.

- You are feeling cranky, helpless, and sad far more frequently.

- You are becoming angry and even a little resentful towards the person you are caring for.

- Your quality of sleep is being impacted.

FINDING STRENGTH IN NUMBERS: BUILDING YOUR SUPPORT NETWORK

- You constantly feel lethargic and you are falling ill more frequently than usual.

Once you have recognized that it is high time to request some help, you need to be mindful of how to ask for it. Remember, you are asking them to take on a difficult and daunting task, and although they will more than likely be happy to help be mindful that how you present your request is more important than asking for it in the first place. Keep these tips in mind next time you reach out to your friends, family, or neighbors for help:

- **Don't ask on a whim plan ahead and communicate your need for help in advance:** Remember, these people have lives too and have other commitments to uphold so they won't always be available to help immediately. For instance, ask your friend on Monday if they will be available to help out with your loved one on Thursday.

- **Describe the situation to them:** For instance, "I haven't slept in days and I have a really important presentation on Thursday that I can't miss, do you think you could watch Mom on Thursday for a couple of hours?"

- **Be specific in your requests for help:** Specify the kind of assistance you need, whether it's someone to watch your loved one while you run errands or someone to help with house chores. Clear and specific requests can make it easier for others to step in and help.

- **Divide the workload:** If you have asked more than one person for assistance, for a particular day, make a list of the tasks you need help with and distribute them among those who agreed to help.

- **Be Realistic:** Be mindful of what a person can and is willing to help you with. If they work a full-time job, avoid asking them to help during the week unless it is urgent

- **Be Flexible:** If they say they can help on Thursday but not on Friday, then try and work with their schedule, not yours.

Don't forget to show appreciation for the support you receive; this will help foster a positive and supportive relationship for future assistance.

CHAPTER 9
MAKING CENTS OF IT ALL—TACKLING FINANCIAL CHALLENGES OF DEMENTIA CARE

Dementia can also be difficult in terms of finances. As caregivers, it is important that we fully comprehend the financial implications that come with caring for our loved ones with dementia. We will explore these financial intricacies that come with dementia caregiving as well as provide you with valuable insights on how you can effectively prepare for these expenses that you will accrue.

Furthermore, we will identify various avenues of financial aid and support by shedding light on these resources that we can utilize to reduce the economic and fiscal strain that caregivers and family members will need to take on. Beyond this, we will be armed with practical tips and strategies for managing financial factors that come with the territory of dementia caregiving, such as medical insurance. By the end of this financial journey, you will be equipped with the knowledge you need to make informed decisions regarding the financial aspects of care.

THE COST OF CARING: UNDERSTANDING FINANCIAL IMPLICATIONS OF DEMENTIA CARE

The Alzheimer's Association's 2023 Alzheimer's Disease Facts and Figures report indicates that family members and unpaid caregivers contribute nearly $340 billion annually to dementia care (Samuels, 2023).

The financial implications of dementia caregiving are bountiful and can often feel extremely overwhelming when you first realize the expenses involved, especially for those who are new to caregiving with no prior experience. Thus, it is essential to have a clear understanding of the most common and anticipated costs you can expect to accrue throughout the caregiving journey so you can both prepare yourself for them and put plans into action before the expenses start piling up.

These costs are expensive and cover a wide spectrum of variables, such as medical treatments, medication, regular doctor appointments, professional caregiving services, home safety modification, and indirect costs such as loss of income due to taking time off work. While most of these are continuous expenses like medication and doctor appointments, some will be once-off expenses, such as modifying your home to be safer.

In-home professional Caregiving

In 2021, it was found that 77% of elderly individuals wanted to age graciously in their own homes; however, dementia can often complicate this decision, especially as their condition progresses (Samuels, 2023). However, if you choose to opt for in-home care, it is immensely beneficial as it can help create an environment that is familiar, safe, and engaging for them. The issue often arises from a financial standpoint, as an average US family can spend over $2000 per month on in-home dementia care.

In-home dementia care costs can vary greatly due to your location and the level of caregiving expertise; thus, you must do your research first. According to Genworth Financial, the average hourly rate for in-home caregivers is approximately $27; however, it can significantly fluctuate. In West Virginia, the hourly rate is $19, while in Minnesota, that rate can be as high as $36 an hour. Keep in mind that if you hire specialized dementia-trained caregivers, you will pay slightly higher rates, with an average of $2.50 more per hour due to the unique skill set required. Thus, it is essential that you assess exactly what your loved ones need and realistically set expectations before selecting a professional in-home caregiver (Samuels, 2023).

Home Modifications

As dementia progresses to its later stages, your loved ones' condition will intensify, leading to challenges such as disorientation, mobility issues, and wandering. By making the necessary modifications to your home to make it safer for your loved ones, you will prevent potential falls and other injury hazards. This could lead to long-term care or hospitalization, which will significantly add to the already overwhelming cost of dementia caregiving. In the early stages of dementia, you will only need to make minor adjustments to your home, such as eliminating trip hazards, adding grab bars, and leveling thresholds, which can mitigate the safety risks associated with dementia and are generally cost-effective. However, as their condition worsens, more drastic and costly modifications may become necessary, such as alarmed windows, doors to prevent wandering, automatic-off appliances, and stair lifts to aid mobility. According to Fixr's 2021 remodeling cost analysis report, dementia home modifications can cost around $9500 (Samuels, 2023).

Medical Expenses

This kind of expense equates to regular doctor appointments, addressing concurrent health complications such as vision problems, hearing loss, and therapy, as well as medication expenses.

The silver lining here is that initial costs, such as diagnostic assessments, are typically covered by comprehensive insurance; however, other experimental treatments and many medications are not covered and will require you to pay out of your own pocket in many cases.

Medicare is the national health insurance that individuals over the age of 65 are eligible for, and it will generally cover the costs of wellness visits, inpatient hospital care, a portion of doctor fees, and health assessments. In 2019, it was found that individual Medicare costs for dementia care were $25,213, which is three times higher than elderly individuals without dementia. As Medicare expenses rise, overall dementia care costs also increase (Samuels, 2023).

Medication Costs

It was highlighted in a Consumer Reports study that monthly costs for dementia medication can fall between the range of $177 and $400+ a month; on the contrary, the Alzheimer's Association indicates a slightly lower cost of $3000 a year, which would be equivalent to $250 a month. It is important to note that these costs would be relevant to your loved ones' unique needs and the dementia stage that they are in (Stringfellow, 2018).

Indirect Costs

Many modern caregivers belong to the "sandwich generation." What this means is that they are supporting their elderly family members in addition to raising children of their own. A report from the National Alliance for Caregiving found that nearly 75% of caregivers who belong to the sandwich generation still hold down a full-time job of their own. What this essentially means is that they dedicate three or more hours every weekday to caring for their loved ones over and above trying to work their normal 40-hour work weeks. This equates to approximately 21 hours a week of unpaid caregiving and often results in them being unable to effectively work for the 40 hours a week of their full-time job, leading to a loss of income (Samuels, 2023).

EXPLORING AVENUES FOR AID: UNDERSTANDING AND ACCESSING FINANCIAL ASSISTANCE PROGRAMS

It's completely natural to feel overwhelmed with all these figures, often unfathomable, swirling around in the back of your mind. You may be asking yourself, "How will my family be able to take on these costs?" If you are asking yourself this question, relax. You can take a deep breath, as luckily, numerous avenues for financial assistance can help financially support you and your loved one through this difficult time. These government, NGO, and private financial aids are in place to help ease the financial strain off of your shoulders

For instance, non-profit organizations like the Alzheimer's Foundation of America offer grants for families affected by dementia. The Alzheimer's Foundation of America offers semi-annual membership grants that will provide you and your loved one with financial support in the form of care assistance, educational resources, and support services to individuals living with dementia, their families, and their caregivers across the US. Each one of these grants provides financial aid in the amount of $6000. They provide these grants twice a year, so that equates to $12000 of financial aid (AFA, 2023).

Medicare is another avenue of financial aid that can help ease the strain of financial expenses. Medicare offers caregivers and their loved ones 100% free nursing home care for 20 days and an additional 80% off for 80 days after that, equating to 100 days of nursing coverage (Burns, 2023). However, Medicare does not include financial aid for custodial care, assisted living, or in-home health aid (National Council on Aging, 2015). Thus, it is often wise to pair up Medicare with another avenue of financial aid known as Medigap. Medigap will help you cover the remaining 20% of nursing home care once your 20-day limit of 100% coverage has expired (AARP, 2023).

Veterans can also benefit from financial support. While the VA may not operate exclusively as a dementia-specific program, it does offer wonderful assistance that can help you weather the storm of looming dementia care expenses with programs like Aid and Attendance. This program provides veterans with anywhere from $1400 to $2100 per month based on their dependents and whether they are married or single, in addition to VA Respite Care, which can help pay for in-home care support (Veteran Aid, 2023).

Medicaid is another invaluable financial aid program for caregivers who need highly skilled dementia care. This federal program typically helps those with low incomes and limited assets cover long-term care expenses. Eligibility may involve a three-year financial review to prevent asset transfers below cost from qualifying for Medicaid (Fay, 2019). Bear in mind that qualifying for this type of support can be quite complex, especially if your loved one has assets, and will often require you to acquire the expertise of a Medicaid specialist or even an elder care attorney. However, your efforts will be well rewarded once you qualify, as Medicaid will cover the costs of nursing home and other long-term care expenses at approved facilities.

These programs can greatly reduce the continual expenses that pile up during the caregiving journey and can provide crucial support for you, your loved one, and your entire family.

MANAGING MEDICAL INSURANCE: NAVIGATING COVERAGE, CLAIMS, AND MORE

Another avenue to reduce the rising costs of dementia care is to understand and effectively manage your loved ones' medical insurance. The first step here is to know their medical aid, like the back of your hand. Make sure you fully comprehend what treatments and services are covered so you can avoid any unexpected expenses in the future. If you happen to notice that a specific service or treatment isn't being covered and you believe it to be a necessary preventative measure, consider exploring other similar covers to see if they can provide what you require in addition to comparable benefits.

Navigating insurance claims is an intricate matter; however, to make this process simpler for yourself, maintaining organization and persistence are key to ensuring that your loved ones receive all their entitled benefits. Make sure you keep an organized record of every medical appointment, treatment, and interaction you have with your medical insurance provider, as this will help streamline the claim process and make it significantly easier for you to track down any expenses for the entitled reimbursements they owe you.

If claims are denied, do not panic. Many claims are initially denied but can often be overruled by being persistent with the appeal process. As I mentioned, being meticulous with keeping a record of all documents, medical records, doctor visits, healthcare provider statements, and any other supporting documentation is vitally important, as this can also help strengthen your case in the appeal process.

Remember to be calm and do not lose your cool when you are dealing with the insurance provider. Engage with them to understand the reason for your claim being denied, and work diligently to get the original verdict overruled in the appeal process. This persistence often pays off, and you will reap the rewards of lightening the financial burden of dementia care expenses and ensuring your loved ones are receiving the quality care they deserve.

PLANNING AHEAD: PREPARING FOR LONG-TERM FINANCIAL RESPONSIBILITIES

Planning for financial expenses is vital in the realm of caregiving. This will help secure the overall well-being of your loved ones and will also give you peace of mind that measures are in place to deal with the anticipated and unforeseen expenses that will accrue throughout the dementia journey. There are several important considerations that you should keep in mind along your caregiving journey to help you navigate the intricate financial aspect of dementia care.

Long-Term Care Insurance

This kind of insurance can be a saving grace for any caregiver, as it can subsidize a myriad of associated dementia costs. The most common expenses long-term care insurance will help cover include paying for in-home services and bearing the brunt of care facility expenses. These are some of the most costly expenses of dementia care, so having this insurance in place can greatly reduce the financial strain of dementia. However, you must do your research before you lock yourself into one of these policies. It would be wise to find one that aligns best with your loved ones' needs and financial situation.

Keep in mind that you need to act swiftly because once your loved one has been diagnosed with dementia, it is extremely unlikely you will be able to apply for long-term insurance coverage. Thus, be proactive and take out this cover before your loved ones have even been diagnosed. If you already have one of these policies in place, it is important to carefully examine the policy and seek answers to several important questions (Alzheimer's Association, 2022):

1. Find out what it covers: Most policies do claim to cover dementia and Alzheimer's disease, but don't take this at face value; instead, thoroughly read through the policy and highlight any specific terms and conditions that are related to dementia coverage.

2. Understand when your loved one can collect their benefits: The majority of policies out there will only trigger benefit payments once your loved one has been medically defined as physically or cognitively impaired; however, make sure you understand this clause thoroughly.

3. Understand what the daily benefits and inflation adjustments are: Understand the exact figure of daily benefits your loved one is entitled to, in addition to finding out if these benefits will be adjusted annually due to inflation. Understanding this will provide you with a clearer picture of the policy's overall value over time.

4. Find out the duration of benefit payments: Some policies stipulate a maximum period of benefit payouts. Therefore, it is wise to inquire from your insurer about the exact duration for which benefits will be paid out.

5. Inquire if this is a maximum lifetime payout policy: Assess the policy to find out whether or not there is a lifetime payout cap on the total amount that can be paid out.

6. Explore the types of care the policy covers: This could include anything from trained nursing home care, subsidized assisted living, adult day care centers, respite care, or other types of dementia-assisted care.

7. Determine the elimination period of the policy: Ask when the insurance will start paying benefits after your loved one is diagnosed.

8. Tax Implications: Check to see if the policy has any tax repercussions because some long-term care insurance benefits may have tax ramifications that you should be aware of.

Reviewing these key aspects of your long-term insurance policy is crucial to ensuring that you completely understand what is stipulated in your loved ones' policy and that you are aware of all aspects of care and financial support they are entitled to.

Legal Documents

Having sound legal documents, such as a living will or power of attorney, in place is crucial to ensuring that your loved ones' financial wishes are respected. This entails drafting a thorough will that lists their assets and preferred method of distribution (National Institute of Aging, 2017).

A power of attorney also gives a trusted person the ability to handle financial matters for individuals living with dementia when their condition has progressed to a stage that limits their capability to do so on their own (Alzheimer's Society, 2019a).

Seek professional guidance

Experts in dealing with the specific financial issues brought on by aging and cognitive decline include elder law attorneys and financial planners. They can provide you with professional guidance to help you make choices that protect your loved one's financial security.

How to Find These Professionals

To identify trustworthy specialists, take into account utilizing on-line resources like the Financial Planning Association and the National Academy of Elder Law Attorneys. These websites can put you in contact with local experts who have the expertise to deal with the tricky economic challenges of dementia care.

By being proactive and making informed financial preparations to ease the stress of dementia expenses, you will have the peace of mind of knowing that those you love dearly will receive the finest care available without financially crippling them.

CHAPTER 10
SAFEGUARDING THE JOURNEY: LEGAL GUIDE TO DEMENTIA CARE

The legal side of dementia caregiving is often a neglected aspect of our roles; however, it holds immense weight in both importance and responsibility. I will equip you with a comprehensive understanding of common legal challenges that arise throughout the dementia caregiving journey by providing you with practical insights on how we can effectively navigate through this legal labyrinth. An in-depth and thorough understanding of the legal realm of dementia is essential to ensuring that both the well-being and autonomy of our loved ones are preserved and respected.

THE CORNERSTONES: POWER OF ATTORNEY AND GUARDIANSHIP

Two factors become important when it comes to the legal responsibilities of your loved one. These two pillars are known as power of attorney and guardianship. They are both legal mechanisms that are essential to ensure the protection of their wishes and, overall, as they gradually succumb to cognitive degeneration, which limits their ability to make crucial decisions on their own. The more we understand these vital legal cornerstones, the better we will be at navigating the legal complexities of dementia with clarity and confidence.

Power of Attorney

This is an essential legal document that should be put in place sooner than later. The purpose of a power of attorney is to essentially grant an individual that you trust, known as the agent or attorney, the full authority to make decisions on behalf of another individual who is unable to make these decisions on their own; this is known as the principal. In this case, the cognitively degenerative nature of dementia would be the reason for the principal being incapable of making sound decisions for themselves. It is wise to make these preparations as soon as possible after their diagnosis, as the National Institutes of Health (NIH) advises individuals to create a power of attorney while their loved ones still possess the cognitive capacity to comprehend the full implications of what this legal document entails. By putting this document in place early on in the dementia process, you are ensuring that your loved ones' wishes and best interests are adhered to and will be upheld as they progress through the various stages of dementia (National Institute of Aging, 2017).

Furthermore, the American Bar Association (ABA) states that it is imperative to select an agent (the individual you are granting authority to) that you trust wholeheartedly. The relationship between the agent and the principal must be built on a foundation of complete trust. This is because an agent wields immense power over the autonomy of the principal and can make both financial and healthcare decisions on behalf of the principal, signifying the immense weight of influence they hold. Selecting an agent you trust will ensure that your loved one's best interests and overall well-being will be protected (American Bar Association, 2013).

Guardianship

Guardianship, on the other hand, is when your loved one is not capable of making sound decisions on their own but has created a Power of Attorney document or appointed a designated agent to make decisions on their behalf. In this situation, the legal system may step in and appoint a legal guardian for your loved one, who will now wield the same power as an agent would with a power of attorney. According to the National Academy of Elder Law Attorneys, guardianship is both a lengthy and costly process, which could potentially involve court hearings and evaluations if the situation requires so (NAELA, 2023).

Guardianship may become necessary when there is no other means of ensuring the individual's welfare and protection; however, practically, a power of attorney is far more ideal if you are in the position to put one in place. Keep in mind that the AARP's Public Policy Institute stipulates that guardianship should be considered your last resort. This is because guardianship can essentially strip your loved ones' rights away from them and eliminate any sense of autonomy they hold (Hahn, 2023).

Consider Having Both in Place

In some circumstances, having a POA and guardianship at the same time can provide a safety net for unanticipated events in dementia care. To determine the best course of action, it is always best to speak with an attorney who specializes in elder law and dementia cases. The proper management of the person's financial, medical, and personal affairs can be ensured by this dual approach, giving everyone involved more security and assurance.

It is important to recognize that legal advice and careful planning are crucial in the process of making informed decisions that both respect your loved ones' wishes and protect their overall well-being.

ADVANCE DIRECTIVES: ENSURING THE PERSON'S WISHES ARE RESPECTED

Like a Power of Attorney or Guardianship, advance directives are vitally important legal documents that hold the power to articulate your loved ones' healthcare preferences and wishes when they no longer can make sound decisions for themselves. The National Institute on Aging stipulates that advanced directives are paramount as they serve as steadfast protectors of your loved ones' wishes and that they will not only be preserved but also respected.

Advanced directives come in many forms; however, the most common documents that make up these directives include a living will, a durable power of attorney for healthcare decisions, and a Do Not Resuscitate clause (National Institute of Aging, 2017).

- A living will is a document that records all of your loved ones' wishes about any medical treatments nearing the end of their lives. Additionally, a living will comes into play when they are permanently unconscious, like in a coma, or completely incapacitated and cannot make decisions for themselves regarding emergency treatment.

- A durable power of attorney for health care is a legal document that will designate an individual, often referred to as a proxy or agent, to make any decisions relating to healthcare for another individual in the event they can no longer make decisions for themselves.

- A do not resuscitate order is when your loved ones have stipulated in their living will that they do not want healthcare professionals to perform cardiopulmonary resuscitation (CPR) if their heart stops or they can no longer breathe. A do-not-resuscitate clause will be placed in your loved ones' medical charts upon being signed off by their doctor.

Advanced directives are imperative to have in place, as they act as guiding lights in the face of medical uncertainty. They provide direction and clarity for all involved, such as healthcare workers and family members.

Discussing and Documenting Preferences In Accordance To Advance Directives

It is paramount to include your loved ones in all discussions regarding their care preferences, as long as their mental capacity allows this to be a possibility. Thus, you must start organizing these documents as soon as possible. Engaging in early and open conversations with your loved ones about their healthcare preferences will be immensely beneficial. This is because it will foster mutual understanding with all involved and ensure their wishes are upheld and respected in the future, in addition to reducing the risk of potential confusion, tension, and conflict as their dementia progresses.

The Mayo Clinic highlights the importance of accurate and thorough documentation of your loved one's preferences in a living will or similar document as their condition worsens.

Documentation is crucial to ensuring that the decisions made by healthcare professionals are aligned with the values and desires of those you care for. Therefore, ensure all their wishes are met and respected (Mayo Clinic, 2020).

Regularly Reviewing and Updating

Bear in mind that advance directives are not static or once-off documents; rather, they require ongoing review. It is advised to continually update these documents so that they remain true and reflective of your love wishes as they evolve.

The National Institute on Aging advises individuals, particularly caregivers and family members, to be diligent and review these legal documents at least once a year. This signifies the importance of revisiting these documents whenever a significant change arises in your loved one's overall health status or progression with dementia (National Institute of Aging, 2017).

Hospitals and healthcare professionals might ask for an original copy of these documents; therefore, you must know exactly where you can locate these legal documents at any given moment. Thus, keep copies and originals in safe and easily accessible locations. According to the National Hospice and Palliative Care Organization, it is advised to keep an organized file with both the original and a copy of these documents, as well as keep diligent notes as to where you can find these documents. This will facilitate swift access in emergencies (Harvard Medical School, 2015).

In essence, ensuring that your loved ones desired preferences coincide with their medical journey even when they are no longer able to be involved in decision-making is an essential part of thorough healthcare planning.

NAVIGATING ETHICAL DILEMMAS IN DEMENTIA CARE

Numerous ethical challenges come with the responsibility of dementia caregiving, and as time passes, these challenges become more pronounced. This is because those living with dementia will find it increasingly difficult to make sound decisions for themselves as dementia progresses to later stages due to their hampered ability to effectively express themselves and make informed decisions based on logic and reasoning.

The Alzheimer's Society stresses that ethics in the realm of dementia caregiving cannot be overstated. They highlight that upholding ethics holds the utmost importance regarding honoring the rights and dignities of our loved ones while still making decisions in their best interest to safeguard their health (Alzheimer's Society, 2021a). Ethics becomes a balancing act of protecting our loved ones while respecting their right to autonomy and dignity. Finding this delicate balance is the key to making effective and ethical decisions on behalf of our loved ones. However, this responsibility is not solely placed on the shoulders of the caregiver. Rather, it is a collaborative effort that requires healthcare professionals and caregivers to evaluate every major decision with sensitivity, respecting personhood, and acknowledging inherent worth as top priorities when making these decisions for your loved ones.

Informed consent is one of the most common ethical dilemmas that caregivers and healthcare professionals may face throughout your loved one's dementia journey. This comes into play when your loved one lacks the cognitive capacity to issue informed consent for medical treatment or to take part as a research participant. In situations like these, healthcare professionals or researchers must obtain clear, informed consent from their loved ones' legal representatives (Alzheimer's Society, 2022). In most cases, this would be the agent or guardian that was appointed in the Power of Attorney or by the court and is generally a family member an individual trusts dearly. Thus, by obtaining informed consent from individuals living with dementia, we can ensure that all decisions made on their behalf will align with their previously expressed values and wishes.

However, it is important to understand that making decisions on behalf of our loved ones is not ideal and should be our last resort, due to the immense power over their autonomy you will wield. Before we start making life-changing decisions on behalf of those we love, we should consider the following to ensure whether or not it is time to take on that kind of responsibility (Alzheimer's Society, 2021a):

- Memory challenges do not necessarily constitute an individual being declared as legally unable to make informed decisions for themselves

- Before resorting to making decisions on behalf of your loved ones, try to make use of tools to aid the decision-making process, such as written notes or voice recorders. These tools are effective in helping support their memories and record their decisions.

- Every human being has the right to receive support to assist them in making decisions on their own until it has been determined they do not have the mental capacity to do this anymore.

- Making decisions completely on behalf of somebody else should not be the solution until various forms of support have been tried and tested to assist them in making their own decisions. However, if supporting their decision has proven to be unsuccessful on multiple occasions, it may be time to step in.

- If necessary, a healthcare professional will conduct tests and assessments to determine your loved one's decision-making capacity. Keep in mind that these evaluations differ across states, so it's best to contact your local Alzheimer's Society for details on your region's regulations.

Furthermore, as our loved ones edge closer to the final stage of their lives, the need for end-of-life decisions becomes increasingly paramount and poses an array of emotional and ethical challenges. When making end-of-life decisions, always try to make them as closely aligned with your loved ones previously expressed values and wishes.

As your loved ones reach the conclusive stage of dementia, it is vital to consider advanced care planning and palliative care. However, it is wise to have an open and frank discussion about their end-of-life preferences while they are still in a position to do so. This discussion will provide you with invaluable foresight that will ensure that their wishes will be respected once they lose their capacity to effectively express them. Palliative care becomes increasingly important near the end stages of dementia. It is a type of care that prioritizes comfort and relief from suffering and is designed to preserve the dignity and quality of life of an individual

In the event of contentious or complex ethical dilemmas, it is always a good idea to consult a healthcare ethics committee for advice on the situation. These committees are entirely made up of experts who can provide you with invaluable guidance and insights to make the decision process smoother, more ethical, and aligned with your loved ones' wishes while still ensuring their well-being is protected.

RESOURCES FOR LEGAL HELP AND ADVICE

Navigating the intricate legal nature of caregiving alone can be extremely daunting, and often we have no idea where to even begin. Thus, obtaining professional legal advice becomes essential. Obtaining advice on legal matters within this domain could involve consulting with a qualified legal professional for guidance. There are resources out there that can make this pursuit easier. For instance, the National Academy of Elder Law Attorneys can assist you in your search to find some of the best elder law attorneys out there. Another resource you can consider is the Legal Service Corporation, which offers free legal counsel to individuals who qualify for this service, such as the elderly or those with limited financial means.

However, before approaching an attorney, organization is key. To prepare for legal advice, compile a list with all your questions and concerns, as this will help facilitate a much smoother and more productive consultation. Furthermore, consider gathering all the documents you need first, such as medical records, financial statements, and any other documents you feel will provide insight for your attorney. You can find a list of what you need, as recommended by the Legal Aid Society, to ensure a more productive consultation.

Lastly, while not a substitute for professional legal advice, online resources can provide a foundation of information and guidance for legal dementia care. Websites like LawHelp.org and ElderLawAnswers offer a wealth of information through articles, guides, and FAQs that can help guide you as you navigate the legal side of caregiving. In addition, when managing insurance claims and medical bills, information from the Federal Trade Commission on consumer protection and rights can be extremely beneficial.

CHAPTER 11
FAREWELL, BUT NOT GOODBYE: NAVIGATING THE JOURNEY BEYOND CAREGIVING

In the complex world of caregiving, one of the most profound emotions we may face is grief. Grief is often overshadowed by the daily demands of dementia caregiving but is a factor of the job that we cannot ignore. As caregivers, we carry the weight of anticipating loss throughout our journey as we watch our loved ones slowly seep away from us as dementia progresses.

Therefore, it is important that we investigate techniques to cope with grief, learn how to hold on to cherished memories, and navigate what lies next after our roles as caregivers.

We will explore how to deal with grief, cherish memories, and navigate life beyond caregiving. We'll learn how heartbreak breeds resilience and how lasting relationships may transcend beyond the conclusive stage of dementia. This chapter is designed to prepare us to find light amidst profound loss.

UNDERSTANDING GRIEF: IT'S MORE THAN JUST SADNESS

It is crucial to understand that grief is an extremely complex emotion and a response to loss that is far greater than the simple notion of sadness. It is an emotion that is multifaceted and deeply rooted in our personal experiences and is triggered when we lose someone we cherish. Essentially, grief is the culmination of vast emotions, each telling a unique story of loss, love, remembrance, and acceptance of what has passed.

Grief presents itself in many forms: the death of those we love, the disbandment of a relationship, anticipated loss, and even losing our jobs. Grief is far more complex than mere sorrow, and due to this, it can often become challenging to understand and navigate on our own.

The Kubler-Ross Model, which is more commonly referred to as the "five stages of grief" helps us understand the grieving process. These five stages consist of denial, anger, bargaining, depression, and finally acceptance. This model is often used to help us comprehend grief through a roadmap, indicating that there is a defined process that we all go through when we experience grief and loss. However, while this model has been effective in helping us understand the concept of grief and its tumultuous terrain, we should not blindly follow this model. This model states that there is a defined journey of grief; however, grief is experienced differently among different people, so we must recognize that grief is not a defined linear journey but a personal journey that takes unique forms in all of us. For instance, people may experience the stages of grief in different orders and may even skip some stages altogether. On the other hand, some individuals may revisit some steps more than once throughout their journey of grief (Psycom, 2022).

Keep in mind that grief is not limited to an emotional spectrum, as this complex emotion can often manifest itself physically affecting our health and well-being. This is due to the extreme stress and painful shock of losing someone we love so dearly. This can take a damaging toll on our bodies. When this happens, it is known as "broken heart syndrome," or its more technical term, stress cardiomyopathy. According to a Harvard study, this condition disrupts the normal pumping function of our hearts and can present similar symptoms to those of a heart. Broken Heart Syndrome serves as a reminder of the link between our emotional and physical health (Harvard Health Publishing, 2018).

Remember, when dealing with grief, it is vital that we listen to what our bodies require and that we prioritize our self-care. Grief has many bodily responses, such as lack of sleep, a decreased appetite, and even a compromised immune system. These symptoms are our bodies signaling inner distress and turmoil, urging us to look after our overall health during these trying times.

Therefore, we need to remember that while the five stages of grief are a framework to help us understand grief, they are not a defined or prescribed path we all adhere to. It is pivotal that while we are experiencing grief as a result of loss, we prioritize self-care and seek support when needed, as we are not alone in this journey.

COPING WITH GRIEF: STRATEGIES FOR HEALING

As we find ourselves in the grieving process, we can often find it extremely challenging to navigate and understand exactly how we are supposed to react. We often feel lost as we have no idea how to manage the emotions we are experiencing; however, grief is an emotion at the end of the day and is just another journey in life we all have to face. Luckily, there are various strategies we can implement to make this process less grueling for ourselves. Just as we have developed coping mechanisms to overcome other challenges in our lives, we can do the same during the bereavement process. Below are some techniques you can utilize to help cope with loss (Three Oaks Hospice, 2021):

- **Don't be afraid to share your feelings:** Confiding in friends and family can help you work through the emotions you are feeling. This does not necessarily mean you are looking for solutions; rather, you are seeking to express your emotions and reminisce about those you have lost with somebody you trust and love.

- **Journal:** Jotting down your thoughts and emotions is a fantastic way to unload what you are feeling on paper. This will help you progress through the mourning stage and keep a record of all your thoughts if you ever wish to revisit them. This is a form of reflection and highlights how your perspective evolves throughout your grieving journey. Remember, grieving is an ongoing journey.

- **Let your creative juices flow:** Activities such as art, music, dancing, writing, crafting, and other creative activities have been proven to improve your overall mood and soften the somberness of bereavement (HSE, 2022).

- **Allow yourself time to grieve:** Allocate specific times throughout the day to be vulnerable and work through what you are feeling. Grant yourself permission to feel whatever emotions you are feeling and express them in your own space free of judgment, whether that be through shouting, crying, punching a bag, or any other emotional release.

- **Don't make drastic life changes:** You are already dealing with a significant loss in your life, so it is wise to maintain a level of stability and familiarity until you have fully gone through the grieving process

- **Avoid isolating yourself too much:** Rejecting social interaction regularly while you are grieving can lead to your emotional response to grief intensifying. Allow yourself to socialize with friends and family every once in a while during these trying times

- **Make time for exercise:** Exercise can help release unwanted emotional energy that is weighing you down. This doesn't need to be an intense workout; it could be a walk or a run around your neighborhood just to clear your head. You could also punch a punching bag if you are dealing with pent-up rage.

- **Allow yourself to remember the good times:** Cherished memories can be a great source of comfort. It can be beneficial to revisit old photos of your loved ones, read old messages they sent you, or even write a letter directed to them. This will help you maintain a connection with those you love even after death.

- **Joining a grief support group:** It can be comforting to share your grief with people who have experienced similar losses. There may also be specialized local support groups for people who have lost a loved one to dementia in your local neighborhood or city.

Grief has no one-size-fits-all approach; each journey is unique. Resilience is common after loss, and feeling okay is perfectly acceptable. There's no need to feel guilty for not conforming to any specific way of grieving.

HONORING YOUR LOVED ONE'S MEMORY: KEEPING THEIR SPIRIT ALIVE

Our loved ones may be gone, but they will never be forgotten. By honoring their memories, we will forever be perpetuating their spirit and the beautiful legacy they have left behind. We can achieve this by creating lasting memories that will last for many years to come, such as planting a tree in their honor or crafting a collage or photo album housing all the precious moments we shared with them. These provide tangible connections that will reinforce their lasting legacy for ourselves and future generations to find solace in. Alternatively, we can keep their spirit alive through charitable donations in their name or volunteering for causes and charities that they hold dear to their hearts. This will channel their undying dedication into action towards communities and causes that matter most to them. Furthermore, in doing this, we are carrying forward their values and passions, ensuring that their impact endures for generations to come (Pathways Health, 2020).

Sharing stories about those we have lost also holds profound therapeutic properties for us. Research has indicated that bereaved individuals who openly engage in storytelling and find solace in their loved ones' memories experience decreased grief and depression, in addition to experiencing a significantly increased overall positive mood. Thus, storytelling is a fantastic way to keep the memories of those we hold dear alive, foster connections even after they have passed, and provide a coping mechanism to enhance our mental well-being (LinkedIn Oral Communication, 2023).

Through these thoughtful acts of honoring those whom we have lost, we are awarded the opportunity to find solace and the assurance that those we care about are still very much alive in our hearts, minds, and actions.

MOVING FORWARD: FINDING A NEW SENSE OF PURPOSE

It is not uncommon to feel like a piece of our very existence has been snatched away from us when our loved ones pass. Often, this leaves a gaping hole that we find immensely challenging to fill. However, amidst this looming emptiness, there are opportunities for us to renew a new sense of purpose for ourselves.

This could come in the form of engaging in a new pursuit, picking up a new hobby, or rekindling our inner fire with a profound sense of commitment and self-achievement. As hard as it is to lose our loved ones, life must go on, and with their passing comes a new dawn of opportunity to chase our dreams and aspirations, thus creating a new reality for ourselves. By finding this new sense of purpose, our loved ones can look down on us and wish us nothing but prosperity and fulfillment in our new journey in life.

What's more, we need to grant ourselves permission to embrace joy and move forward with our lives. Life does go on, and we owe it to ourselves and those we love to be resilient and forge a new path. We need to understand that even if we experience joy during the grieving process, it does not signify in the slightest that we have forgotten about those we cherish or that we are not grieving appropriately. Rather, we should view it as a testament to the natural evolution of healing and the beauty of personal growth, as time heals all wounds. For some, healing comes sooner than others.

Purpose comes in many shapes and sizes. Engaging in volunteer programs or community activities has profound psychological and healing benefits. It fosters a meaningful connection with others and can elevate our mental well-being, in addition to strengthening our feelings of social belonging.

As the sun sets, a sunrise will follow. Discovering happiness again after loss becomes a crucial element in honoring the memory of those we hold so dear and helps fulfill their desires as they can rest easy knowing your well-being is protected. Joy after grief signifies the remarkable resilience of the human spirit and shows to the world that one can always find the light even amid grief's shadows.

SHARE YOUR EXPERIENCE WITH ANOTHER CAREGIVER

Did you know that the most beautiful gifts in life are those that we give without expecting anything in return? That's something I've learned on this journey of caregiving, and have been blessed to share it with you.

If you have gained anything from these pages, please consider leaving a review for this book.

Please use the link below to share your thoughts:

[https://www.amazon.com/review/review-your-purchases/?asin=B0CW1K34ZX]

Thank you from the deepest part of my heart. I hope you have enjoyed this book and it has helped you even is some small way. May your journey continue to be blessed!

With gratitude,

Mary Ann Martin

SHARE YOUR EXPERIENCE WITH ANOTHER CAREGIVER

AFTERWORD

Our journey through the world of dementia care has been marked with compassion, empathy, insight, understanding, wisdom, and a deeply human experience. From the beginning, we've walked hand in hand through this journey as we delved into the intricate and complex realm of dementia. We explored the many aspects of this degenerative condition, traversing through its many stages, and shed light on its unmistakable symptoms This knowledge formed the foundation of our understanding and acted as a beacon that will ultimately help us be more empathetic and effective as we care for our loved ones.

With this foundation in place, we proceeded to equip ourselves with the tools and knowledge we needed to close the communication gap between ourselves and medical professionals, deepen our understanding of dementia through highlighting its common treatments, break down communication barriers with our loved ones, and identify the significance of familiarity and routine when caring for our relatives with dementia. These crucial pillars helped us become better caregivers for both ourselves and our loved

AFTERWORD

ones. Today, we are in a position to navigate the ever-evolving and complex challenges that dementia presents daily.

However, our journey did not end there. While comprehensively understanding dementia and how to become a more effective caregiver is essential, understanding the continual rollercoaster of emotions that caregivers deal with internally is just as crucial to understand and manage. We unearthed strategies to help us cope when the responsibility of caregiving becomes too overwhelming and arduous. We focused on the strength that we have within us and learned why self-care is necessary. Remember, it is okay to share the load to avoid caregiver burnout and prioritize your health every once in a while without grappling with feelings of guilt. Our journey has reinforced that it's natural to experience a spectrum; however, there are many avenues to find solace and reassurance, even in difficult times.

Furthermore, we delve even deeper, considering factors of caregiving that are often overshadowed by more immediate issues. However, we were proactive and explored the complex financial and legal aspects of dementia care. With this knowledge, we were able to plan for the future and have peace of mind that future challenges would be taken care of. Through anticipating future challenges, we confidently charted our course for this caregiving journey, securing the best possible care for our loved ones and preserving their dignity when the need for more drastic measures arises.

Lastly, we have prepared ourselves for the inevitable and highlighted the importance of maintaining equilibrium. We explored the importance of grieving, honoring our loved ones after death, and finding purpose in ourselves once we set forth on our path in life after our roles as caregivers. Understanding this is a poignant reminder that life is comprised of many chapters, and caregiving is only one of those chapters.

Don't forget that you are never alone in your journey. Seek out guidance from support groups, where you'll receive invaluable guidance and mutually beneficial experiences. Investigate professional care services, financial aid, and legal guidance using the advice found in this guide. Keep sharpening your skills as a caregiver, as every challenge that you will face in your life provides you with the opportunity to grow and improve as an individual.

Never abandon your courage and fortitude. Your effort extends far beyond executing mere tasks; it is a tribute to your compassion, love, and the profound impact you have had on the lives of those you cherish. Remain optimistic as the everlasting force of love defines your journey. You possess the power to navigate through life's triumphs and tribulations with a heart filled with joy, grace, and adorned humility. Always remember love, and you will leave a legacy behind that will be cherished and remembered for a lifetime.

GLOSSARY

1. **Advance Directive:** A Legal document that states a person's healthcare preferences in the event of incapacitation.

2. **Agnosia:** When a person is unable to recognize or identify people or objects

3. **Aphasia:** a language disorder that affects an individual's ability to communicate effectively due to dementia.

4. **Cholinesterase Inhibitors:** A categorized group of medications that are used to help improve cognitive function in dementia patients

5. **Caregiver Burnout:** Physical, emotional, and mental exhaustion experienced by caregivers.

6. **Cerebrospinal Fluid Analysis:** A medical exam, executed through a lumbar puncture, is used to detect abnormal proteins linked to specific dementias like Alzheimer's.

7. **Cognitive Decline:** Decrease in cognitive abilities, such as memory and thinking skills.

GLOSSARY

8. **Computed Tomography (CT) Scan:** This is a type of scan that can quickly detect structural issues in the brain and can detect issues like dementia, tumors, or strokes.

9. **Delirium:** A state of severe confusion and disorientation, it can happen suddenly without any warning

10. **Magnetic Resonance Imaging (MRI) Scan:** Scans that offer high-detail brain structure information, including region-specific atrophy (a decrease in size of a body part or tissue), and aids in diagnosing various forms of dementia

11. **Memantine:** A drug class used to treat individuals who are diagnosed with mid-stage and late-stage dementia. It regulates glutamate - a crucial brain chemical that facilitates memory and learning.

12. **Mild Cognitive Impairment (MCI):** This is the stage between normal-age appropriate cognitive degeneration and more severe dementia symptoms

13. **Neurodegeneration:** Is the progressive loss of nerve cells, a common feature in most types of dementia.

14. **Neurologist:** A physician specializing in the nervous system, including dementia.

15. **Neurofibrillary Tangles:** When dementia patients' brains have unusually twisted fibers

16. **Palliative Care:** Specialized medical attention aimed at lessening symptoms and raising patients' quality of life who suffer from dementia.

17. **Positron Emission Tomography (PET) Scan:** This scan is used to assess the brain metabolism and beta-amyloid plaques (a clump of proteins on the brain), aiding in diagnosing and tracking dementia

GLOSSARY

18. Respite Care: Temporary relief for caregivers, providing them a break from caregiving duties.

19. Sundowning: Increased confusion and agitation in the late afternoon and evening.

20. Wandering: Patients with dementia frequently wander aimlessly and in a potentially hazardous manner.

BIBLIOGRAPHY

AARP. (2023, January 20). *What is medicare supplement insurance, aka medigap?* AARP; AARP. https://www.aarp.org/health/medicare-qa-tool/what-is-medigap-insurance.html

AFA. (2023). *Grant information*. Alzheimer's Foundation of America. https://alzfdn.org/find-a-member/grant-information/#:~:text=Our%20Bi%2DAnnual%20membership%20grants

Alzheimer's Association. (2019). *Medication safety*. Alzheimer's disease and dementia. https://www.alz.org/help-support/caregiving/safety/medication-safety

Alzheimer's Association. (2022). *Stages of Alzheimer's*. Alzheimer's Disease and dementia; Alzheimer's Association. https://www.alz.org/alzheimers-dementia/stages

Alzheimer's Association. (2023). *On the front lines: Primary care physicians and Alzheimer's care in America*. https://www.alz.org/media/Documents/alzheimers-facts-and-figures.pdf

Alzheimer's Association. (2019a). *10 early signs and symptoms of Alzheimer's*. Alzheimer's Disease and Dementia; Alzheimer's Association. https://www.alz.org/alzheimers-dementia/10_signs

Alzheimer's Association. (2019b). *Wandering*. Alzheimer's Disease and Dementia. https://www.alz.org/help-support/caregiving/stages-behaviors/wandering

Alzheimer's Association. (2022). *Insurance*. Alzheimer's Disease and Dementia. https://www.alz.org/help-support/caregiving/financial-legal-planning/insurance

Alzheimer's Association. (2023). *Caregiver stress*. Alzheimer's Disease and Dementia. https://www.alz.org/help-support/caregiving/caregiver-health/caregiver-stress#:~:text=Find%20time%20for%20yourself.

Alzheimer's Association. (2022, October 19). *Eating and dieting*. Alzheimer's Association. https://www.alz.org/media/documents/alzheimers-dementia-eating-ts.pdf

Alzheimer's Disease International. (2023, March 12). *ADI - Dementia statistics*. Alzheimer's Disease International. https://www.alzint.org/about/dementia-facts-figures/dementia-statistics/#:~:text=Numbers%20of%20people%20with%20dementia

Alzheimer's Society. (2018). *Positive language -Style guidelines Positive language An Alzheimer's Society guide to talking about dementia*.

BIBLIOGRAPHY

https://www.alzheimers.org.uk/sites/default/files/2018-09/Positive%20language%20guide_0.pdf#:~:text=For%20those%20living%20with%20dementia

Alzheimer's Society. (2019a). *Lasting power of attorney*. Alzheimer's Society. https://www.alzheimers.org.uk/get-support/legal-financial/lasting-power-attorney

Alzheimer's Society. (2019b, July 15). *Reducing caregiver stress*. Alzheimer Society of Canada. https://alzheimer.ca/en/help-support/im-caring-person-living-dementia/looking-after-yourself/reducing-caregiver-stress

Alzheimer's Society. (2020, June 17). *Can caring for a pet help a person with dementia?* | *Alzheimer's Society*. Www.alzheimers.org.uk. https://www.alzheimers.org.uk/blog/can-caring-for-a-pet-help-a-person-with-dementia#:~:text=Animal%2Dassisted%20interventions%20can%20improve

Alzheimer's Society. (2021a). *Dementia and decision-making*. https://alzheimer.ca/sites/default/files/documents/Conversation-About-Decision-Making-en-Alzheimer-Society.pdf

Alzheimer's Society. (2021b, September 30). *Sundowning and dementia*. Alzheimer's Society. https://www.alzheimers.org.uk/about-dementia/symptoms-and-diagnosis/symptoms/sundowning#:~:text=The%20reasons%20why%20sundowning%20happens

Alzheimer's Society. (2022). *Consent and capacity of people with dementia*. Alzheimer's Society. https://www.alzheimers.org.uk/dementia-professionals/dementia-experience-toolkit/how-recruit-people-dementia/consent-and-capacity

Alzheimer's Society . (2021, August 14). *Daily care of teeth*. Alzheimer's Society. https://www.alzheimers.org.uk/get-support/daily-living/daily-care-teeth#:~:text=Generally%2C%20the%20easiest%20way%20is

Alzheimer's (2022, November 15). *Finding dementia care and local services* . National Institute on Aging. https://www.alzheimers.gov/life-with-dementia/find-local-services

American Bar Association. (2013). *Power of attorney*. American Bar https://www.americanbar.org/groups/real_property_trust_estate/resources/estate_planning/power_of_attorney/

American Family Physician . (2018). Prescribing Cholinesterase Inhibitors for Alzheimer Disease: Timing Matters. *American Family Physician, 97*(11), 700–700. https://www.aafp.org/pubs/afp/issues/2018/0601/p700.html#:~:text=The%20most%20common%20adverse%20effects

Berg-Weger, M., & Stewart, D. B. (2017). Non-pharmacologic interventions for people with Dementia. *Missouri Medicine, 114*(2), 116–119. https://www.ncbi.nlm.nih.gov/pmc/articles/PMC6140014/

BIBLIOGRAPHY

Betsaida, A. (2018, June 22). *Aromatherapy for dementia*. News Medical. https://www.news-medical.net/health/Aromatherapy-for-Dementia.aspx#:~:text=Benefits%20of%20Aromatherapy%20for%20Dementia&text=It%20has%20been%20widely%20used

Boston University. (2021, March 8). *Music as a memory tool for patients with Alzheimer's*. Chobanian & Avedisian School of Medicine. Boston University. https://www.bumc.bu.edu/camed/2012/12/12/music-as-a-memory-tool-for-patients-with-alzheimers/#:~:text=Researchers%20found%20that%20general%20content

Bristal, T. (2021, January 21). *11 Essential questions Alzheimer's caregivers should ask a doctor*. The Bristal. https://blog.thebristal.com/11-essential-questions-alzheimers-caregivers-should-ask-a-doctor

Brown, M. (2023, April 25). *Dealing with caregiver guilt*. Caregiver. https://caregiver.com/articles/dealing-caregiver-guilt/#:~:text=Recognize%20your%20strengths%20and%20don

Burns, J. (2023, August 29). *Does medicare pay for nursing home care?* Fortune Well. https://fortune.com/well/article/does-medicare-pay-for-nursing-home/

Daily Caring . (2023, January 18). *8 benefits of caregiver support groups*. DailyCaring. https://dailycaring.com/8-benefits-of-caregiver-support-groups/#:~:text=How%20caregiver%20support%20groups%20can

Dementia Australia. (2014a). *What is dementia?* Dementia Australia. https://www.dementia.org.au/about-dementia/what-is-dementia

Dementia Australia. (2014b, August 4). *Frontotemporal dementia*. Dementia Australia. https://www.dementia.org.au/information/about-dementia/types-of-dementia/frontotemporal-dementia

Dementia Australia. (2014c, August 4). *Lewy Body Disease*. Dementia Australia. https://www.dementia.org.au/about-dementia/types-of-dementia/lewy-body-disease

Dementia Australia. (2014d, August 8). *Tests used in diagnosing dementia*. Dementia Australia. https://www.dementia.org.au/national/about-dementia/how-can-i-find-out-more/tests-used-in-diagnosing-dementia

Dementia Australia. (2015a). *Vascular dementia*. Dementia Australia. https://www.dementia.org.au/about-dementia/types-of-dementia/vascular-dementia

Dementia Australia. (2015b). *Physical exercise and dementia Can physical exercise reduce the risk of developing dementia? Can physical exercise help people with dementia?* https://www.dementia.org.au/sites/default/files/helpsheets/Helpsheet-DementiaQandA08-PhysicalExercise_english.pdf

Dementia Australia. (2022). *Alzheimer's disease*. Dementia Australia. https://www.dementia.org.au/about-dementia/types-of-dementia/alzheimers-disease

BIBLIOGRAPHY

Dementia Australia . (2023, April 18). *Types of dementia*. Dementia Australia. https://www.dementia.org.au/information/about-dementia/types-of-dementia#:~:text=We%20now%20know%20dementia%20is

Department of Health & Human Services. (2019). *Dementia - hygiene*. Better Health. https://www.betterhealth.vic.gov.au/health/conditionsandtreatments/dementia-hygiene#hair-care-and-dementia

Family Caregiver Alliance. (2016). *Caregiver statistics: Demographics*. Family Caregiver Alliance. https://www.caregiver.org/resource/caregiver-statistics-demographics/

Fay, B. (2019). *Financial help for Alzheimer's caregivers & dementia patients*. Debt. https://www.debt.org/medical/financial-help-alzheimers-dementia/

Hahn, S. (2023, March 8). *Rethinking guardianship*. North Carolina. https://states.aarp.org/north-carolina/rethinking-guardianship

Harvard Health Publishing. (2018, April 2). *Takotsubo cardiomyopathy (broken-heart syndrome) - Harvard Health*. https://www.health.harvard.edu/heart-health/takotsubo-cardiomyopathy-broken-heart-syndrome

Harvard Medical School. (2015, June 6). *Keep your living will safe but accessible*. Harvard Health. https://www.health.harvard.edu/staying-healthy/keep-your-advance-directive-safe-but-accessible#:~:text=Hospitals%20may%20request%20an%20original

Harvard University. (2022, July 15). *Diet Review: MIND Diet*. The Nutrition Source. https://www.hsph.harvard.edu/nutritionsource/healthy-weight/diet-reviews/mind-diet/

Hoy, T. (2021, October). *Support groups: Types, benefits, and what to expect*. Help Guide. Https://Www.helpguide.org. https://www.helpguide.org/articles/therapy-medication/support-groups.htm

HSE. (2022, September 2). *Improve your mood by doing something creative*. HSE. https://www2.hse.ie/mental-health/self-help/activities/doing-something-creative/#:~:text=Doing%20something%20creative%20can%20help

Kwon, O.-Y., Ahn, H. S., Kim, H. J., & Park, K.-W. (2017). Effectiveness of cognitive behavioral therapy for caregivers of people with dementia: a systematic review and meta-analysis *Journal of Clinical Neurology, 13*(4), 394. https://doi.org/10.3988/jcn.2017.13.4.394

LinkedIn Oral Communication. (2023). *How can storytelling help clients cope with trauma and stress?* Linkedin. https://www.linkedin.com/advice/1/how-can-storytelling-help-clients-cope-trauma#:~:text=Storytelling%20can%20help%20you%20cope%20with%20trauma%20and%20stress%20by

Logan, B. (2016). *Caregiver's guide to understanding dementia behaviors*. Family Caregiver Alliance. https://www.caregiver.org/resource/caregivers-guide-understanding-dementia-behaviors/

Mayo Clinic. (2019a). *How Alzheimer's drugs help manage symptoms*. Mayo Clinic. https://www.mayoclinic.org/diseases-conditions/alzheimers-

BIBLIOGRAPHY

disease/in-depth/alzheimers/art-20048103

Mayo Clinic. (2019b, December 1). *Memantine (Oral Route) side effects*. Mayo Clinic. https://www.mayoclinic.org/drugs-supplements/memantine-oral-route/side-effects/drg-20067012?p=1

Mayo Clinic. (2021, August 8). *How to choose the right support group*. Mayo Clinic. https://www.mayoclinic.org/healthy-lifestyle/stress-management/in-depth/support-groups/art-20044655#:~:text=Support%20groups%20bring%20together%20people

Mayo Clinic . (2020, August 22). *Your guide to living wills and other advance directives*. Mayo Clinic. https://www.mayoclinic.org/healthy-lifestyle/consumer-health/in-depth/living-wills/art-20046303

NAELA. (2023). *Guardianship and conservatorship*. NAELA. https://www.naela.org/Web/web/consumers_tab/consumers_library/consumer_brochures/law_topics/guardianship_conservatorship.aspx

National Council on Aging. (2015). *National council on aging (NCOA)*. NCOA. https://www.ncoa.org/

National Institute of Aging. (2017). *Staying physically active with Alzheimer's*. National Institute on Aging. https://www.nia.nih.gov/health/staying-physically-active-alzheimers

National Institute of Aging . (2017). *Legal and financial planning for people with Alzheimer's*. National Institute on Aging. https://www.nia.nih.gov/health/legal-and-financial-planning-people-alzheimers

National Institute of Health. (2015, June 2). *Studies show benefits of caregiver support programs*. National Institutes of Health (NIH). https://www.nih.gov/news-events/nih-research-matters/studies-show-benefits-caregiver-support-programs

NHS. (2023, August 18). *Communicating with someone with dementia*. NHS. https://www.nhs.uk/conditions/dementia/living-with-dementia/communication/

Pathways Health. (2020, February 12). *Is it ok to be happy during grief? | Pathways*. Pathways Home Health and Hospice. https://pathwayshealth.org/grief-support/is-it-ok-to-be-happy-during-grief/

Physiopedia. (2010). *Informed consent with people who have dementia*. Physiopedia. https://www.physio-pedia.com/Informed_Consent_With_People_Who_Have_Dementia

Psycom. (2022, June 7). *The five stages of grief*. Psycom. https://www.psycom.net/stages-of-grief

Ralph-Savage, M. (2020, October 13). *The value of positive language when caring for someone with dementia*. Relish Life. https://relish-life.com/blog/the-value-of-positive-language-when-caring-for-someone-with-dementia

Robinson, L. (2022, February 2). *Volunteering and its Surprising Benefits*. Help Guide. Https://Www.helpguide.org. https://www.helpguide.org/arti-

BIBLIOGRAPHY

cles/healthy-living/volunteering-and-its-surprising-benefits.htm#:~:text=Volunteering%20provides%20many%20benefits%20to

Samuels, C. (2023, June 13). *Surprising costs of dementia care.* Www.aplaceformom.com. https://www.aplaceformom.com/caregiver-resources/articles/cost-of-dementia-care#medical-cost-of-alzheimers-care

Stringfellow, A. (2018, June 28). *Dementia care costs by state: An overview of costs, types of dementia care, and the cost of dementia care by State.* Caregiver Support and Resources. https://careforth.com/blog/dementia-care-costs-by-state-an-overview-of-costs-types-of-dementia-care-and-the-cost-of-dementia-care-by-state#:~:text=Dementia%20-Care%20Levels%20%26%20Their%20Associated%20-Costs&text=For%20example%2C%20a%20Consumer%20Reports

The University of Texas. (2020, November 3). *How much of communication Is nonverbal? | UT Permian Basin Online.* The University of Texas. https://online.utpb.edu/about-us/articles/communication/how-much-of-communication-is-nonverbal/#:~:text=The%2055%2F38%2F7%20Formula&text=He%20found%20that%20communication%20is

Three Oaks Hospice. (2021, April 6). *Bereavement strategies - Coping with grief and loss.* Three Oaks Hospice. https://www.threeoakshospice.com/blog/bereavement-strategies-coping-with-grief-loss/

Veteran Aid. (2023). *Alzheimers and dementia care.* Veteran Aid. https://www.veteranaid.org/alzheimers-demnetia.php

Watson, S. (2022, January 11). *Caregiving help: Ask for what you need.* WebMD. https://www.webmd.com/alzheimers/alzheimers-caregiving-help

WebMD. (2001, September 4). *Recognizing caregiver burnout.* WebMD. https://www.webmd.com/healthy-aging/caregiver-recognizing-burnout

Where you live matters . (2020, July 27). *Why Is Routine Important for Dementia? | Where You Live Matters.* ASHA. https://www.whereyoulivematters.org/importance-of-routines-for-dementia/

World Health Organization. (2023). *Dementia.* World Health Organization. https://www.who.int/news-room/fact-sheets/detail/dementia

Printed in Great Britain
by Amazon